BEYOND THE
MASTER
CLEANSE

BEYOND THE MASTER CLEANSE

The Year-Round Plan
for Maximizing the Benefits
of **The Lemonade Diet**

Tom Woloshyn

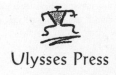

Ulysses Press

Published by: Ulysses Press
P.O. Box 3440
Berkeley, CA 94703
www.ulyssespress.com

ISBN: 978-1-56975-690-4
Library of Congress Control Number: 2008907000

Printed in the United States by Bang Printing

10 9 8 7 6 5 4 3 2 1

Acquisitions Editor: Nicholas Denton-Brown
Managing Editor: Claire Chun
Editor: Keith Riegert
Copyeditor: Elyce Petker
Proofreader: Emma Silvers
Production: Judith Metzener
Index: Sayre Van Young
Front cover design: what!design @ whatweb.com
Cover photo: ©istockphoto.com/Susan Trigg

Distributed by Publishers Group West

"MASTER CLEANSE" is used in the title and contents of this book in its generic
sense as a term for a detoxification diet that has been widely used and discussed
since it was first introduced in 1941. This book is an independent work of information and commentary and is not affiliated with, or sponsored or endorsed by,
any manufacturer of consumables or other goods and services.

NOTE TO READERS
This book has been written and published strictly for informational and
educational purposes only. It is not intended to serve as medical advice or to be
any form of medical treatment. You should always consult your physician before
altering or changing any aspect of your medical treatment and/or undertaking a
diet regimen, including the Master Cleanse diet as described in this book. Do not
stop or change any prescription medications without the guidance and advice of
your physician. Any use of the information in this book is made on the reader's
good judgment after consulting with his or her physician and is the reader's sole
responsibility. This book is not intended to diagnose or treat any medical
condition and is not a substitute for a physician.

To my friend, Robert Veal Jr.

Contents

What Is the Master Cleanse?

The Master Cleanse is a ten-day liquid mono-diet of fresh-squeezed lemons, maple syrup and cayenne pepper designed to enhance and assist your body's natural ability to cleanse and detoxify itself. Created by my mentor Stanley Burroughs in 1941, this simple regimen has been used by millions of people worldwide with inspiring results. Since my first cleanse in 1979, I have personally spent over 1,000 days on the diet and have successfully guided thousands of others through their own Master Cleanse experiences.

My first book, *The Complete Master Cleanse*, delves into the specific properties, correct procedure and remarkable effects and benefits of the Master Cleanse—explaining simply and concisely how it works. Unfortunately, I have found that nearly half the people I talk to who have attempted the Master Cleanse without correct guidance have done it incorrectly. My goal with *The Complete Master Cleanse* was to help people avoid the perils, pitfalls and even pain of attempting the Master Cleanse without proper help. After all, the Master Cleanse brings remarkable changes in your life—from increased energy and clarity of mind to less aches and pains, from weight loss and improved skin to the healing of troubling health disorders; in fact, my former wife conquered cervical cancer with the help of the Master Cleanse!

In addition to reviewing the correct way to approach the Master Cleanse, this book will show you how to maintain the cleanse's amazing health benefits so that you are not sliding back into an unhealthy lifestyle and continually in need of rigorous cleansing. This book will help give your lifestyle a kick start and develop a long-term strategy for healthier eating habits, future cleansing and a brand new approach to life in general.

From my 29 years as a holistic health practitioner and consultant, I have learned to identify the most common trouble spots people encounter in their lives post-Master Cleanse. In the following chapters I hope to give a better understanding and offer insights as to why you may be experiencing continuing pain or health challenges and how to start overcoming them. From my experience, identifying and properly addressing these problems early can reduce the need for continual cleansing. In this book you'll find invaluable information to help you improve both your physical and mental health, from easy parasite cleansing and avoiding common toxins to overcoming addictions and transitioning to a new diet.

Successfully completing the Master Cleanse is a great accomplishment! But now you may turn your attention to your broader future and continue your transformation for the years to come. You've already taken one challenge head-on; this is your chance to live a happier, healthier and more prosperous, abundant life!

PART ONE

The Master Cleanse in Review

If you have not already done your Master Cleanse, this section will serve as a primer to help guide you through the ten days of diet transformation. However, for more in-depth instruction and information, you should use my first book, *The Complete Master Cleanse*.

Benefits of the Cleanse

Over my many years of practice, people have reported myriad benefits that occur during or after a Master Cleanse. To give only the principal ones:

Better sleep—It is deeper and more restful.

More energy—Those who complete the cleanse experience increased energy to the point where some people start following an exercise program, even though they have never exercised in their lives.

Clarity of mind—People tell me that a burst of awareness has come over them, almost frightening them, because after a cleanse they realize how out of touch they were with their bodies and their overall health.

Positive outlook—One woman called me on Day 37 to thank me for my help with her cleanse, because she no longer harbored thoughts of suicide.

Greater flexibility—Even yoga instructors who have done a cleanse have told me how astonished they were at their increased physical flexibility.

Weight loss—Women often lose one pound per day during a cleanse, men up to two pounds.

Freedom from addictions—I have known many people who stop smoking, using alcohol, doing recreational drugs or consuming junk foods.

Increased strength—During and after a cleanse, many people who like to work out are able to increase their weight load when at the gym.

Pain and swelling—These conditions are often reduced.

Hair loss—People report their hair stops falling out and increases in body.

Better skin—Problem skin clears up and becomes healthier.

Reduced allergies—Some allergies are significantly lessened, and others can even disappear entirely after a cleanse or two.

You may experience many more positive outcomes from doing the Master Cleanse!

First, mentally prepare yourself for the cleanse and all that it involves. Be aware that whenever people start a Master Cleanse on a whim, they tend to go off it on a whim. It lacks importance to them, so it's no wonder they fail on it. Therefore, it's best to set a goal of at least ten days on the Master Cleanse. Set those days aside and make sure you don't have a full calendar of social events. It usually is best not to tell too many people (or sometimes anyone outside your own home) that you are doing a cleanse.

Second, do not let others discourage you. I have seen many prospective cleanses aborted by third-party doubters and skeptics who have never themselves done the Master Cleanse or who, if they have done it, did it incorrectly. Do not let others sabotage your efforts. You'll want to surround yourself with people who support you in your journey toward greater wellness.

How to Get Started

Some people like to prepare their body before a cleanse. They go on a primarily vegetarian diet for four or five days, then ramp up to an all-veggie diet before starting the cleanse itself. This simpler diet will be less stressful on the body and will help with the eventual elimination of some of your poor food choices. Eating such a diet will make it easier for you to transition to the Master Cleanse.

If you drink coffee or caffeinated soda every day, you will want to prevent the headaches that are caused by caffeine withdrawal. Start taking pantothenic acid (vitamin B-5) for about four days before starting the cleanse. The dosage should be approximately 400 mg., taken three times a day, while at the same time you reduce your coffee or soda intake about 25 percent each day. This will help you taper off the caffeine that you are accustomed to having. The day you start your cleanse, you will be off coffee or soda completely and will no longer need to take the vitamin supplement.

Most importantly, you will need to go out and gather your ingredients: lemons, maple syrup, cayenne pepper, herbal laxatives and sea salt. (See the sections below for full details and properties of all ingredients.) If you have no other source of good water, you will need to add bottled water to your list. Whenever possible, buy organic lemons to make your lemonade drink; it will taste much better and will also have a higher nutritional quality, since it won't have been treated by pesticides, herbicides or chemical fertilizers that are typically used in commercially grown produce. Some consumers might complain about the higher cost of organic produce, but remember that this is the only food you will be eating for ten days or more—so get the best; you deserve it.

Contraindications and Cautions

People who have had organ transplants and are on immune-suppressant drugs *cannot* do the Master Cleanse. The cleanse will stimulate the immune system and also inhibit the effectiveness of the drugs, a combination that will likely cause the immune system to attack the transplanted organ and end in serious—and possibly dangerous—problems.

I believe that most drugs are acid forming in the body. I do know that drugs should not be flushed down the toilet or thrown in the garbage because they are considered toxic. Unused medication should be returned to the pharmacy.

Issues with Lemons or Cayenne

The Master Cleanse uses lemons and cayenne, precisely because they possess properties that are good for stirring up toxicity in the body. Their effects, however, are often mislabeled or misunderstood. If you are already somewhat toxic and you are eating either lemons or cayenne or both and experiencing discomfort or what you think is an allergic reaction, this may be due to your body's simultaneous attempt to cleanse itself *and* digest food. This creates a conflict; sometimes it even causes severe discomfort. When you are on the Master Cleanse you are not eating any other foods, so the issue of other food allergies does not arise.

Surrender to the Process

It can be hard to try something entirely new, especially if it's something that sounds a bit weird or even risky—even though you hear good things about it from people you trust. You might try this little mental exercise that I often give to clients who are anxious. At first glance it seems odd, but it works:

1. *Know where you are.* Imagine that you have called a travel agent and are asking her to book you a flight, but you have no idea where you are! This is a disconcerting feeling, so avoid it by taking the time to center yourself.

2. *Know where you are going.* Again call the travel agent and say, "I am in Seattle but I don't want to go to New York or Miami, not to Atlanta, either. I also don't like London as a destination." The agent, in frustration, will ask, "Well, where *do* you want to go?"

3. *Surrender to the process.* You know where you are and where you want to go. You now have to trust the travel agent, the airline, the taxi driver, the baggage handler, and all concerned that they will get you and your suitcase to your destination. The agent will ask for the dates you want to travel and for payment. Your only responsibility is to show up at the airport at the right time on the proper day, and as if by magic you will soon arrive at your destination. You do not have to design the plane, build, fuel or fly it. *You just get on the plane!* You surrender to the process that others have established and tested.

Now apply this exercise to your current state of health and the goals you desire to achieve by using the Master Cleanse. Start by surveying your present state of health. Once you know where you are, move on to the next step—defining the results you want.

As you think about your first Master Cleanse, be flexible and open-minded about it, just as you would if you were flying overseas for the first time and feeling a little anxious. In both situations you could meet a little turbulence or have to change flights partway there, or be bothered a bit by rough weather. Just trust yourself and be willing to roll with whatever comes up.

Don't get upset or disturbed if every little thing doesn't happen exactly the way you might expect. This process can be exciting and adventurous. This journey toward better health may change your life—it will almost surely bring you much more than you imagine.

It just so happens that I am writing this paragraph on the exact day when, 27 years ago, I was taking a course on Stanley Burroughs's work. Did I know that that first step would start me on the long road to where I am today? No, but I did know it was absolutely the thing I wanted to do—so I surrendered myself to doing it with a happy heart.

How to Do the Master Cleanse

Again, while this section of the book is a helpful tool for doing the Master Cleanse, it is geared more toward increasing your health *after* the cleanse. You should read *The Complete Master Cleanse* from cover to cover to ensure absolute success on your first Master Cleanse. Make notes or highlight steps, cautions and tips you feel are especially helpful.

Make sure you understand how to do the Master Cleanse properly so that you can complete it with success and experience the benefits. I'm amused to recall that Stanley Burroughs would often say something that technical support people still tell their frustrated customers: "WAEFFTI—When All Else Fails, Follow The Instructions."

GOOD TO READ

Some readers might profit from browsing through Stanley Burroughs's original small volume, *Healing for the Age of Enlightenment*. The author self-published it in 1976; it was revised and reprinted in 1993. Though the book is sometimes out of print, a limited number of copies may be available through used bookstores or an online book vendor.

Follow these steps, in order (they are explained at length in the sections below).

1. Gather the ingredients.

2. Take an herbal laxative the night before you start the cleanse.

3. The next morning, repeat the laxative or drink an internal salt water bath.

4. Be sure to have three or four bowel movements every day while using the laxative.

5. Now start to drink the lemonade, freshly made: six to twelve glasses each day.

Step 1—Gather Ingredients

First, assemble all the ingredients you need to do your cleanse. Buy only enough lemons for about three days at a time if you can. (You will need a total of approximately 60 to 100 lemons, depending on their size, for a ten-day cleanse.) If you wish to use limes instead of lemons, make sure that they are ripe and starting to be yellow in color; a dark green lime is unripe.

A close friend did the Master Cleanse using only green, unripe limes and after several days complained that she felt sick with every glass of limeade she drank. Limes that have developed brown spots become bitter tasting and should not be used.

It is best to keep lemons on a counter at room temperature, or to even set them in the sunlight; this allows them to ripen. I check my lemons and limes once or twice a day to make sure they are not starting to spoil. If they are ripening too quickly, I rub a small amount of lemon essential oil on the lemon or lime peel to prevent spoilage.

Lemons and limes kept in the refrigerator will have a lower enzyme activity (which you don't want) and be less flavorful. If you have refrigerated lemons, remove them about two days before you use them.

Step 2—Take an Herbal Laxative

With the ingredients all assembled, you will begin the Master Cleanse by taking an herbal laxative the night before you start. The laxative may be in the form of a tablet, capsule, or tea. If you prefer tea, make it according to instructions, but make a note of how strong it turns out; it may need to be steeped longer, or to have another tea bag added, to strengthen its effects. When using the laxative in tablet or capsule form, you generally need at least three to five of them to create the desired results.

Whatever the form you take it in, the laxative must be used each and every night of the Master Cleanse. This will ensure that you eliminate all the toxins that your body is releasing.

The laxative may cause diarrhea symptoms in some people. If this occurs, stop taking it until the diarrhea has stopped. Please remember that this is a liquid mono diet, with no fiber whatsoever to bulk up in the colon. The continual ingestion of fluids, combined with the elimination of runny, slimy mucus and old waste, will make your bowel movements appear as though you have diarrhea. (In fact, you do not.) It can take two to three days for the stool to go from firm to rather loose. The diarrhea symptoms I am speaking of are manifested when you have to run repeatedly to the bathroom several times a day without much control of your colon.

Step 3—Repeat the Laxative, or Drink a Salt Water Bath

In the morning of Day 1 of the cleanse, before drinking lemonade, either repeat taking the herbal laxative or use an internal salt water bath. The internal salt water bath is made by adding two teaspoons of noniodized sea salt to one quart of warm water. The salt water is mixed to the same salinity as your blood. When you drink this mixture, the salinity keeps the water from being absorbed into the bloodstream. You will not absorb the salt unless you are deficient in salt or the many trace minerals it contains. The salt water normally passes into the colon and out the rectum.

You can drink the salt water bath every morning, or can omit it completely if you use the laxative instead. (I have taken the internal salt water bath hundreds of times, and I find it pleasant to do.)

There are several considerations to weigh before making your choice. The downside: The salt water bath can start to be eliminated within half an hour, or can take up to one and a half hours to take effect after you drink it. The final elimination of the salt water will often come about one hour after your first elimination.

The upside to the salt water bath is that, with it, you will not have to make any urgent runs to the bathroom throughout the rest of the day. This is very helpful if, for example, you are in a dentist's chair with the dentist's hands in your mouth, in a business meeting during the day or are traveling on an airplane (though you will try to avoid that). Occasionally, someone will not pass the salt water on their initial attempts. If this happens, don't worry about it; just add more salt the next time.

The herbal laxative can cause cramping. This is usually the result of your colon's discharging some rather nasty stuff. At a certain point you will not want to overdo the laxative, because it may cause severe cramping, even nausea. I find that, for me, the laxative is better at eliminating waste from the colon, so I usually do the salt water bath only three times in a ten-day cleanse. I drink the salt water on Day 1, then again on Day 3 or 4, and finally on Day 7 or 8.

Please do *not* drink the quart or liter of salt water all at one time, as you will probably be disgusted with it and throw it up. I take about ten minutes to drink my salt water, and I warm it to body temperature before consuming it. Some people imagine they are drinking a salty soup or broth, which seems to work for them. You may find the salt water distasteful at first, but after a short time you should get used to it and it will become easy to swallow.

Step 4—Have Daily Bowel Movements

It is vital that you have at least three to four eliminations from your bowel each day when you are using the herbal laxative. Some people experience what they colorfully describe as a "ring of fire" during elimination. To be plain about it, this is merely a combination of the cayenne pepper and acidic waste being passed from the bowel.

The best remedy is usually to apply coconut oil on the affected area. (Coconut oil is found in health food stores or in the natural foods section of some supermarkets.) Do not use hand cream or lotion on tender tissues because they usually contain chemicals that are severely irritating.

Step 5—Start Drinking the Lemonade

The first morning and every other morning of the cleanse, you will begin to drink the lemonade when you are hungry (normally within the first hour or two after arising), or, if doing the salt water bath, after you begin eliminating the salt water. Drink six to twelve glasses of lemonade every day. Drink the lemonade whenever you are hungry, and try not to let yourself get overly hungry. Remember that while the Master Cleanse is a simple process, many people create a little difficulty with it. Therefore, please follow instructions carefully.

TIP

To measure cayenne for the lemonade: Use a measuring spoon set. The smallest spoon in the set is usually ⅛ teaspoon; fill it about three-quarters full. Many people find the cayenne hot at first, so you may want to begin with less than ⅒ of a teaspoon and work up to the full amount.

JUICING WITH EASE

Treat yourself to a good-quality electric citrus juicer. Juicers of this type are far more efficient than hand juicers and will produce more juice than if you squeeze by hand or utensil into a glass. You may wish to buy a used juicer in good working order to do your first several Master Cleanses, then move up to a new one of better quality.

Always drink your lemonade fresh. Drink it within ten minutes after you prepare it. Drink it whenever you feel hungry. Start drinking the lemonade about one hour after taking your laxative or after your first elimination of the salt water bath. Drink 6 to 12 glasses a day (each mixture amounting to at least ten fluid ounces).

I suggest that, unless you are obese, you consume at least eight glasses of the lemonade mixture each day. I myself often drink 12 glasses a day, and will drink as many as 16 glasses if I am extremely physically active. I know someone who drank 24 to 26

Mix Your Lemonade

—Place 2 tablespoons of freshly squeezed lemon juice into a glass. (Use a measuring spoon for accuracy.)

—Add 2 tablespoons of maple syrup.

—Add 1/10 teaspoon of cayenne powder.

—Fill the glass with eight ounces of good-quality water.

—Drink up!

---

glasses a day (that is, two gallons!) while training for a triathlon, and did so for 12 days in a row. If you feel hungry, tired or cold, it is often because you are not drinking enough lemonade.

If the lemonade tastes too sweet or you want to lose weight, you can decrease the maple syrup in each drink by half a tablespoon. If you desire to maintain or gain weight, however, you may add half a tablespoon of maple syrup to each drink.

You can alternate drinking water or herbal tea with the lemonade throughout the day. It is important, however, not to drink too much water and not enough lemonade. Drink water or herbal tea if you feel dehydrated or when the weather is hot. Remember, you must drink at least six glasses of lemonade per day!

- Never microwave your lemonade. Doing so will destroy many of its valuable enzymes and vitamins and will diminish its effectiveness.
- Follow these simple steps—to the letter!—and you will most likely succeed by having a good, productive Master Cleanse.

Master Cleanse Ingredients and Their Properties

Maple Syrup

You might be wondering, "Where will I get the energy I need during the cleanse if I eat nothing at all?" The ingredient in the Master Cleanse program that provides you with the fuel for your body over the period of the cleanse is pure maple syrup—plain

> ## A Simple Alternative to Fresh
>
> For those people who cannot make their lemonade fresh for each drink—because they will be away from home—there is a simple alternative. Mix equal parts of maple syrup and lemon juice as a concentrate into a dark container and keep it cool; a thermos is ideal. Prepare enough concentrate to last as long as you will be away. Whenever you hanker for a glass of lemonade, measure four tablespoons of this concentrate into a glass, add the cayenne pepper and the water, stir and drink. The maple syrup will act as a preservative for the lemon juice, which in turn will help to prevent oxidation of the vitamin C and the enzymes. Note that as soon as you add water, you must drink it—say, within five to ten minutes.

and simple. Stanley Burroughs recommended it because of its high quality as a food as well as its general availability. You may use raw cane syrup or freshly pressed cane juice, if available, instead of maple syrup.

Maple syrup's properties are what make it suitable for a cleanse. Maple syrup contains a number of minerals and vitamins in trace amounts. Depending on where the syrup was collected, the amount of nutrients in it varies, as does its taste. Both are determined by mineral content in the soil and the growing conditions of the maple trees. Potassium, calcium, magnesium, manganese, phosphorus, sodium iron, zinc, copper, tin, sulfur and silicon can be found in maple syrup. Vitamins A, B-1, B-2, B-5, B-6, biotin and folic acid are present as well, along with a miniscule amount of amino acids.

Maple syrup is generally marketed in four grades. Some confusion can arise between the old and the current grading system. The old system had A, B, and C grades. The current grading system runs from lightest to darkest: Gr. [Grade] A Light Amber, Gr. A Medium Amber, Gr. A Dark Amber, and finally Gr. B. The problem began with the original system, where Gr. A was considered better than Gr. B and, of course, much better than Gr. C, which led to large differences between the A and B grades in selling price. At times I have seen Gr. A sell for twice the price of Gr.

C, although now all grades sell at roughly the same price. Canadians will need to use #2 Amber grade.

The difference in the grades is a result of the time period in which the sap is collected from the maple trees in the spring. The first run of sap is called Gr. A Light Amber. This consists of sap that the maple tree stores in its roots over the winter. The warm days and cold nights make the sap run up into the tree and will act as antifreeze; it will also feed the tree. The reserves in the roots, as they are used up, urge the roots to absorb moisture from the soil and to continue to pump sap up into the tree. This new uptake of water by the roots brings with it trace minerals from the soil that will darken the sap.

This first run, Gr. A Light Amber, is light in both color and taste, owing to its lack of minerals. During the winter the sap in the roots loses some of its mineral content. The Gr. A Medium Amber is a combination of older, light sap mixed with newer and heavier sap laden with minerals. As the season progresses, the concentration of minerals continues to increase and Gr. A Dark Amber is the next run. The final run of sap, or Gr. B, is all new uptake from the roots and has the highest mineral content. *Gr. B maple syrup* is actually the highest quality syrup for the Master Cleanse and the best possible choice. Stanley recommended Gr. B (or what was called Gr. C); if neither is available, get the darkest grade you can buy. One tablespoon of maple syrup supplies about 55 calories (about 200 per quarter cup).

Other Sugars or Sweeteners You must never substitute any artificial or processed sugar, such as Splenda, Equal, aspartame or others of their ilk for maple syrup.

Agave is another sweetener that is becoming widely available, though it is not a good choice for the Master Cleanse. It is made from the agave plant, which is high in a compound called inulin (or fructosan), which is extracted as a dark juice, filtered to remove minerals and heated to convert the inulin into fructose.

Finally, it is concentrated to make syrup. Usually, two grades of agave juice are available—light and dark.

Fructose is a sugar used extensively by the processed food industry and soda drink manufacturers. It has been made widely available from the production of corn syrup. Fructose has a low glycemic index. This lowered insulin secretion fools the body into not recognizing the caloric intake; this, in turn, blocks the body's ability to regulate food intake or to control weight gain. This missing "feedback loop" makes you consume more foods, which are then converted to...you guessed it, fat.

Any sugar that is good for your health should be produced by a single-stream method of manufacture. This means one product in and only one product out—not multistream, which results in the removal of various amounts of mineral content. This is an extremely important point because it is the natural mineral content whole sugars that make them safe for consumption. (Maple syrup that is 100 percent syrup is "whole" or unadulterated, and therefore safe.)

I have known of a practitioner who restricts his clients' use of agave to only ten days of the cleanse. People doing more than that were found to be suffering from demineralization. It's logical that eating demineralized foods (that is, all processed or whitened foods) causes the body to go into "mineral debt." This results in specific organs being weakened by the lack of proper nutrients, making them unable to function properly or to replicate their cells normally.

If you ever read pirate-and-treasure stories as a youth, you may have heard about the crew that was shipwrecked in the Bahamas while carrying a precious cargo of sugar from Caribbean plantations to the Old World (Europe). A storm forced their ship onto a reef, where it foundered and was about to go down. Some of the crew swam to shore and were able to salvage portions of the cargo. The members of the crew who ate the processed sugar for several days were said to have gone quite crazy, while those who consumed only food scavenged from the island stayed well until they were rescued. Lesson learned?

Glucose and the Pancreas   Your body burns glucose, and only glucose, for fuel. *Everything* that you metabolize as energy comes from glucose created from carbohydrates, proteins or fats. Many people have found themselves to be highly sensitive to sugar from their overconsumption of processed sugars and starches since childhood. This acquired sensitivity can cause them to experience both high and low fluctuations of energy. The sufferers often compensate for these unpleasant feelings by eating even *more* complex carbohydrates, proteins and some fats, thus worsening the cycle.

Complex carbohydrates have a lower glycemic index and raise blood sugars more slowly than do simple sugars, such as pastries or other baked goods using white flour and white sugar. Proteins and fats have to be converted by the liver into sugar; this requires a longer lead time to release sugar into the body and makes for its "more-regular" influx into the bloodstream. This slower and more-regular uptake of fuel by the body enables the pancreas to keep blood sugar levels properly balanced. The problem with this approach is that it is only symptomatic, not causative. My analogy for this: If you accidentally knocked a hole into a wall of your house, would you hang a nice picture over it— or would you repair it?

As you can probably imagine, the new dietary lifestyle that many people follow these days, including eating more complex carbohydrates, is actually only a mask. People think they're doing the right thing and eating the right foods, which indeed they are, on one level. But they have not addressed the root cause. I have seen these people eat fruit and still experience the roller coaster ride of imbalanced sugar levels. Take the picture down off the wall ten years later, and the hole is still there. We should fix the problem at its source, not just give it (so to speak) a "sugar coating."

When a pancreas suffers damage by excessive processed foods and white sugar, it also suffers nutritional deficiencies from the lack of many minerals and vitamins. One job of that organ is to regulate blood sugar levels to within one-tenth of one percent. It now should be obvious to you that devitalized foods and foods devoid of minerals and vitamins do a double whammy on the pancreas. Their lack of nutrients weakens the pancreas, and the dramatic rise in blood sugar levels from the easy absorption of these foods stresses that organ by pushing it to overproduce insulin. This causes the roller coaster highs and lows that many people experience throughout the day, even though they think they're eating "normally."

This rocky ride often stems from childhood. How frequently do you "reward" your own children or grandchildren with a sugar-laced treat or see other parents do so? The child receiving this reward starts to associate love and care with sugar, and at an unconscious level naturally learns to crave it in order to feel good. Why else do you think we call certain foods "comfort food"?

We have made an error of associating certain kinds of foods with love and attention. Just try to watch television while doing the Master Cleanse, and you will be surprised at the food commercials and how they will make you tempted to eat. (I have not consumed hamburgers for decades and I am not normally interested in eating them, but when I am on the cleanse and I happen to see TV ads showing juicy hamburgers I sure do want to eat one.)

Stevia One popular sweetener that many people ask about using on the Master Cleanse is called Stevia, also known as sweetleaf or sugarleaf. This product is not a true sugar but a compound extracted from a very sweet but indigestible herb in the sunflower family. It provides no calories or energy at all for you while you are on the cleanse. Therefore, if you use it, you will be starving yourself—something you do not want to do.

Lemons

Lemon is a unique food, in a class all its own. (A lime is chemically equivalent.) Lemon is an acid food—yet, paradoxically, it is highly alkalizing to the body when digested. The several acids in lemon help to break down various calcified substances throughout the body, such as kidney stones and gallstones. The high levels of potassium, calcium and magnesium found in a lemon makes a lemon an optimal choice to alkalize the body's tissues.

You likely have smelled lemon essence in many cleaning agents, polishes and soaps. Lemon juice is used extensively to clean computer chips in the high-tech industry. Lemon is also a natural cleansing agent for the body's insides since it breaks and loosens mucus to be eliminated. This property has made it a common home remedy for treating colds and flulike symptoms. For example, whenever I feel a cold coming, I drink a glass of lemonade with plenty of cayenne pepper, and usually all my symptoms disappear within an hour or two.

A lemon contains calcium, magnesium, potassium, phosphorus, sodium, zinc, copper, selenium and iron—but there's even more to it than that. Lemon is the only fruit or vegetable that contains more anions than cations. *Anions* are atoms or molecules that carry a negative charge, while *cations* are atoms or molecules that carry a positive charge. This positive (or negative) charge will determine a food's properties when consumed by the body. The anionic quality is much the same as in saliva, bile, the stomach's digestive fluids and digestive enzymes. All of these assist the body in breaking down unhealthy tissues and cells that it then recycles to regenerate itself.

Lemons are high in vitamin C, as you no doubt know. They also contain lesser amounts of thiamine, riboflavin, niacin, pantothenic acid (vitamin B-5) and vitamin B-6. In addition, they contain a small amount of protein and fiber, plus an assortment of other trace nutrients. There are about four insignificant calories per tablespoon of lemon.

Do *not* use Meyer lemons for the Master Cleanse. While these are delicious in baked goods, they are unsuitable for the cleanse because they are less acidic and have slightly different properties. Meyer lemons are considered a cross between a true lemon and a mandarin orange; in southern Texas they are called Valley lemons.

Cayenne Pepper

Herbologists often refer to cayenne as the "master herb." It is typically ground from the pods and seeds of pungent, long, tapering red peppers of the genus *Capsicum*. When mixed with most other herbs, cayenne acts as a catalyst—that is, it makes the other herbs react, and thus work more effectively.

Cayenne pepper is a stimulant that raises metabolism, increases circulation by purifying and thinning the blood and helps many digestive disorders. You might be amazed to learn that, when placed under the tongue as a tincture or powder, cayenne can even stop a heart attack. It will halt internal bleeding, and it can even be applied directly as first aid to external areas of the body that are bleeding.

Like lemon, cayenne breaks up and loosens mucus in the body. This benefits the sinuses, the bronchial tubes and lungs, and it allows clearer and easier breathing. Cayenne is high in both vitamins A and C, and contains some B vitamins as well. It also contains potassium and calcium, both of which make it highly alkalizing to the body.

Capsaicin is the most active compound found in cayenne. It is cayenne's *heat* that we sense in the taste and also by touch (which is why Asian and Mexican chefs wear rubber gloves when handling certain superhot chili peppers). Its heat is what makes cayenne a pain reliever to the body, and it is an ingredient in numerous over-the-counter products and ointments.

A pepper's hotness is measured in Scoville units; cayenne typically ranges from 40,000 to 100,000 on this scale. I suggest that people unfamiliar with cayenne start at the bottom end of the scale. When cayenne pepper is not rated by the packager, it is generally at the 40,000 Scoville units level. Always test the hotness of the cayenne by using a small amount until you become familiar with its properties and its results in your system.

You can purchase cayenne in most supermarkets, usually in the spice section, as well as at organic food stores and health food stores. Purchase cayenne pepper that is deep red or orange. Cayenne fades in color with age and should be stored in a cool, dark place.

Water

In addition to lemon and cayenne, water is another vital component of the Master Cleanse. As fetuses, we spent most of our first nine months suspended in amniotic fluid in the womb; that fluid is mostly water. Our body consists of about 70 percent water, so the need for good water for proper health cannot be overstressed.

Water is the universal solvent and is likely needed universally to support life (one reason that scientists are always trying to find water on other planets or moons). It will dissolve more compounds than any other fluid. This is an important point, because by now you know that the cleanse is designed first to break up, loosen, and dissolve wastes and toxins in the body and then to flush them out.

You probably know that water is used to help flush and transport toxins to the organs of elimination (the colon, bladder, lungs, skin and so on) so that the body can discharge them. Some people believe that many health problems can be significantly improved, or completely eliminated, with just an adequate consumption of good water.

I cannot overstate the importance of using good-quality water during the Master Cleanse. Depending on the source and treatment of your city's water supply, you may have excellent water coming directly out of your tap. A vast number of brands of bottled water can be purchased today in stores and supermarkets, or can be home-delivered; I cannot comment on them or recommend one over another. A few cities still maintain artesian (or deep) wells as free-flowing sources of good water. Water-treatment systems in the home are growing in popularity because of some cities' or counties' questionable quality of tap water. Avoid chlorinated and fluoridated water.

In your cleanse, try to use water that is free of impurities or chemicals added by water treatment facilities. An often overlooked but important quality is water's pH level (its acidity or alkalinity on a scale that ranges from 0 to 14; "pH" stands for "potential of hydrogen"). The Master Cleanse is designed to alkalize your body, so it is most important that you learn the pH level of the water source you will be using. Water for cleansing or drinking is best when the pH level is 7.0 or slightly higher. You can buy an inexpensive water-pH-testing kit (available at most drugstores) to help you determine what water is best for you to drink. Abundant Health is one among many distributors of pH strips (at a cost of about two cents per strip).

In addition to the Master Cleanse program, some people choose to do a water fast. They take in only water for several days or even weeks. Stanley Burroughs, developer of the Master Cleanser, did not believe that people should do a water fast unless they first did the cleansing. When I was practicing in Toronto I treated several individuals who did water fasting regularly before they came to me for treatment. These people said they felt better, had more energy and had significantly better results from the Master Cleanse. I have never water fasted myself, so I cannot make a qualified judgment on the pros and cons of this therapy.

Reverse Osmosis Water Water that is put through reverse osmosis (called RO water) is sometimes used for a Master Cleanse, though it is not ideal for that purpose. Such water goes through a dual-filtration system: First it is filtered through carbon and then through a thin membrane that allows some water to flow through while catching and rejecting most impurities.

This system has one major drawback, in addition to cost: About 75 percent of the water is rejected and dumped down the drain, thereby being wasted. Acidifying the water before it comes to the membrane will make the filter more efficient, thus wasting less water and producing more filtered water. But such acidified water is detrimental to the Master Cleanse and is best *not* to be used.

Distilled Water   Stanley did not recommend using distilled water; he colorfully, if truthfully, said it was "cooked." The distillation process boils off oxygen as it is dissolved and removes many useful trace minerals that are naturally found in the water. Distilled water is also slightly acidic.

If you need to use distilled water, I suggest that you set covered containers of it outside in the sun for two or three days to be recharged. Then add back trace minerals by shaking a few grains of sea salt into it or adding a few drops of a trace mineral supplement in liquid form.

My Own Water Preferences   I use a water ionizer, both for my drinking water and for doing the Master Cleanse. This unit has a carbon-filtration system and uses a process that creates two streams of water—one acid, one alkaline. The alkalinity of the resulting water can be adjusted from about pH 7.0 to 9.0, depending on the acidity of your tap water. Many other treatment systems are available. I have even heard of some good systems that use magnets, though I cannot speak for their efficacy.

I have developed a rather unusual technique to enhance not only the taste but also the quality of the water I drink and use for the Master Cleanse. Suspend your disbelief here, please! I store my water in a one-gallon, covered, glass container that bears the labels *love* and *gratitude*. This may sound strange indeed, but the water simply tastes better after being in a container with those two words.

Abundant Health, a distributor of pH strips for testing water, also sells stick-on, reusable labels that bear a variety of positive words. You can place labels of your choice on your water containers to charge them with the feeling or thought of your choice.

The principles of *homeopathy* are consistent with this water-imprinting work. A homeopathic remedy is made by diluting a medicine in an aqueous solution to such a degree that the original compound is virtually undetectable. This extreme dilution still carries the signature of the concentrated compound in the water. For centuries people throughout the world have used homeopathy. It is becoming increasingly popular as an alternative holistic therapy because some people experience great success with it.

Supplements

You should *not* use supplements while on the Master Cleanse. Such nutrients (whether in pill or liquid form) will stimulate your digestive processes and may even stop the detoxification process—something you do not want to do. The Master Cleanse works effectively, just as I have outlined it.

A few supplements are known to not interfere with the cleansing process and, in fact, to assist the body in healing. Herbs and herbal teas of all types (but without adding anything, such as honey or other sweeteners) can be used with the cleanse. I strongly recommend the use of parasitic remedies (page 59). Digestive enzymes may be used while on the Master Cleanse since they are not a food. These enzymes will assist the lemon and cayenne to break down undigested food and waste that have built up in the colon.

I have taken as many as ten enzyme capsules at a time, three or four times a day, while on the cleanse, and I have noticed an increase in the number and bulk of my eliminations. As always, it is important to use good-quality enzymes; these can be obtained through a number of resources, including most health food stores and many online sites.

Essential Oils   It is acceptable to ingest essential oils for the cleanse since as they do not need to be digested and are already in their simplest form to be used by the body. I take certain essential oils by mouth while on the cleanse. Drops of lemon essential oil can be added to your lemonade, and essential oils can be encapsulated and taken internally.

DO NOT ingest essential oils, however, unless you absolutely know that they are therapeutic grade.

What to Expect During the Master Cleanse

You need to know some of the ups as well as the downs of the Master Cleanse because you will respond differently to the detoxification process than the next person will. While I myself have only had positive experiences with the Master Cleanse, and while I know many people who have had successes similar to mine, a few folks will become troubled by physical or emotional issues that arise during their cleanse.

Over many years of practice and consultation, I have learned that everyone has his or her own unique experience with their first cleanse. I also know that each successive cleanse can be quite different from the first one. About four in ten people may experience headaches, joint pain, low energy and a general feeling of malaise at one or more stages during the cleanse.

This is not at all unusual because your body is going through withdrawal from sugar, caffeine and other addictive foods, while at the same time familiarizing itself with a low-protein liquid diet *and* at the same time stirring up toxic wastes in your body that will be eliminated. These symptoms are, in fact, caused not by the Master Cleanse but by what you have done to your body in the past.

The Master Cleanse is something like a time machine in that it takes you back in time and you re-experience old symptoms or conditions as you stir up the old toxins in your body. These old toxins are stored because of stress. In the same way, the Master Cleanse can free the same emotions and feelings that were left unfinished in some way.

I have had people on the Master Cleanse say they can taste cigarettes in their mouth, yet they have not smoked for many years. People who did recreational drugs years ago sometimes feel high, or "stoned," as old drugs get released from fat cells in the body. I have witnessed people get dilated pupils as they cleanse. One client had done chemotherapy recently and indicated that he was still burping the drugs up after 27 days of being on the cleanse. People will speak of craving foods they have not eaten for ten years or so; the toxins from these foods are now entering the bloodstream and triggering old memories.

In the past, I typically had my clients come in for a consultation and then come back to have a Vita-Flex treatment during the period that they were on the cleanse. During the Vita-Flex treatment, certain points on the feet would be supersensitive to my touch, indicating that a specific area of the body was experiencing a lack of wellness. I would ask if they now have, or have had, a problem in that specific area; sometimes my clients would say, "No, no problems there." About Day 5 or 6 they would call me and tell me that yes, they are having a problem, and "Guess where?" I would patiently explain to them that I could tell there was indeed a problem, but it had not yet surfaced. (Remember that dis-ease starts in the mind and manifests itself in the body.) I would add, maybe a bit smugly, that they were lucky to have caught it before it became a major problem, and together we would tackle the problem and come up with a solution.

You cannot always know what to expect, even when it seems obvious or logical to you. I have treated people who had been given only a week to live, yet after they started the Master Cleanse they would immediately begin feeling better.

I also had a friend who once described himself as "healthy as a horse," though he could not last even one day on the Master Cleanse. Several months later this friend confided in me that his usual regimen, before doing the cleanse, included eating eat five or six chocolate bars each day, apparently without its affecting his health! He seemed oblivious to the amount of caffeine and white sugar he was regularly ingesting—but he felt the consequences when he began the Master Cleanse and couldn't stay on it.

Healing Crisis: A *Good* Thing

The four out of ten people who do the cleanse and have a little trouble with it usually say they have one day in particular that is hardest to get through. They explain that it is not always a physical condition or discomfort that they are feeling. People who facilitate or work with people doing detoxification programs of one sort or another often describe such symptoms as a "healing crisis."

Crises of this type occur when the various organs of elimination are forced to function at an accelerated pace, in order to deal with a sudden influx of wastes from the various tissues in the body. (Think of a flash flood rushing down a bone-dry riverbed.) The symptoms can be really dramatic, but may only last minutes; in some people, they can last several hours or more.

When people I have treated call me to say they are dying, I calmly reply, "No, you're not dying. You are getting better." They protest that idea and again say, "Really, I'm dying!" Of course, I can detect from their intonation that they are just feeling bad, so I assure them that what's happening is that they are getting better—but feeling worse for the moment. These bad feelings often clear up after the person has eliminated. If it continues for more than a day, I suggest to them that they consider doing one or more of Stanley Burroughs's adjunctive therapies, such as Vita-Flex and Color Therapy. After using these therapies some people can, in only minutes, completely alleviate all or most symptoms.

A healing crisis is actually beneficial, though it is often misinterpreted by people and may be the very thing that causes them to halt the cleansing process. Psychotherapists sometimes explain to their patients the distinction between having a mental "breakdown" and experiencing a "breakthrough" in self-awareness and understanding. The same holds true with the physical body.

Menstrual Cycle Changes

Many women to whom I have recommended the Master Cleanse reported that while on the cleanse their menstrual cycle started at a different time of the month than usual. This is a typical reaction. They go on to say that their discharges are often darker and heavier, but only temporarily. I assure them that they need not be concerned about the blood loss on the Master Cleanse.

I have even had clients donate blood while on the cleanse, which has greatly surprised me. (Most people would never consider doing such a thing while on a cleanse.)

Comfort Food

Many people eat comfort food (discussed earlier), which is the consumption of something (usually something unhealthy) to displace emotional discomfort. When the coping mechanism is taken away (that is, they run out of that yummy food or that heavenly drink or that pep-up snack), they feel distressed. But drinking lemonade on the Master Cleanse does not act like your favorite comfort food, nor will it ever replace it. Now, wait: This is not a bad thing. In fact, it creates an opportunity for you to deal with some past experience in a real way so that you can let it go.

I have seen people become angry, sad or confused during the cleanse, as the detoxification process stirs up their feelings. I reassure them that these feelings are like clouds; they will pass, and the sun will shine again. Doing a Master Cleanse can make clear what our emotional relationships with food really are.

Other Conditions During a Cleanse

It is rare but not uncommon to feel *nausea* during the cleanse. The queasy feeling usually disappears after the individual throws up. Most people report that what they vomit is only mucus and that they feel fine afterward. I have known only three or four people whose nausea did not dissipate, even when they tried drinking ginger tea. If the problem persists for more than one day, I suggest that the person stop the cleanse and attempt it again in a week or so. The wait is often all that is needed for the cleanse to work.

You can also expect to have *bad breath,* since you are breathing out toxins from your lungs and your mouth. *Body odor* also becomes worse, because you are excreting toxins through your skin. Your *bowel movements* can smell terribly foul. All of these are not a bad thing—they are better coming out than staying in and continuing to poison your body.

You may also feel your *sinuses* draining and *mucus* loosening in your throat. Your *skin* may worsen for a short time as well. All are indications that these organs have been overloaded in the past and are now letting go of various irritants. Such conditions generally do not last long and are not troubling.

During the cleanse, it is important that you assess your own experience with it and decide whether you wish to continue giving it your very best try. If you experience a *healing crisis* during your cleanse, as described above, you will have to make a judgment as to what to do. At that point you might seek support, use supportive therapies or stop the cleanse and consider trying again at a later date when you feel stronger or more hopeful. (See Resources for some guidance for support.)

Having Problems During the Cleanse?

The Master Cleanse is obviously not a program for everyone. But it isn't always easy to tell in advance whether a given person will take to the cleanse, tolerate it and end up benefiting from it.

I have known many clients and even friends to endure tremendous discomfort and pain, to a degree that I myself would probably not want to put up with. Yet most were highly motivated people who were willing to experience a healing crisis to get to the other side and feel well. For most people the worst day is usually Day 3 of the cleanse. Other common problem days are Days 1 and 4.

Having a problem day occurs about 40 percent of the time, but the number of problems experienced skyrockets if the cleanse is done incorrectly. The most common mistakes are:

—Not drinking the lemonade fresh
—Omitting the laxative
—Not drinking adequate amounts of lemonade

Almost daily I talk to someone on the cleanse who is experiencing problems, and a large percentage of these people are doing it wrong—wrong ingredients, wrong amounts, wrong timing and wrong foods before the cleanse.

My own experience was—and continues to be—very positive and enjoyable. During the time that I was writing my first book, I did the Master Cleanse three times. In all my years of experience, I have never had any healing crises, headaches or pains while on the cleanse. No, wait a minute...I spoke too soon: I do remember that, during my fourth cleanse, I started to get canker sores. This is not at all unusual, as the cleanse is also correcting the tissues in the mouth. After two or three days of sores, someone from my Stanley Burroughs training suggested using a recommendation of his: gargling with a half-and-half mixture of apple cider vinegar and water several times a day. That was all I had to do, and my canker sores completely cleared up.

I attribute my continued success with the cleanse to maintaining a positive attitude about the cleanse and having a clear expectation of its benefits. I tell myself that I deserve to have a good result, and I always get one. Conversely, I have seen people embark on the cleanse with a lot of fear and trepidation, experience some discomfort that they interpret as a problem (and a failure of the Master Cleanse *for them*), and so they stop immediately.

Some people expect the worse—and in fact *feel* worse—in a kind of self-fulfilling prophecy. Yet some of these same people, while doing medical interventions, lose their hair, or get extremely weak, or live in constant pain, or have diarrhea and many more

---

Mind Helps Body Help Mind

On a trip I met a shy young woman. After talking with her, I advised her to read the Burroughs book and try a Master Cleanse. Later, she called me on Day 3 to say she was feeling great and had lots of energy. On Day 7 she phoned to tell me that she had low energy, hated how the drink tasted and wanted to stop. I replied that stopping the cleanse when you're feeling bad is not the best thing to do and assured her that she was going through a healing crisis; her physical symptoms were an expression of a deeper underlying emotion. We spoke for quite a while. Remembering my first impression of how she looked uncomfortable with her appearance, I drew her out about it, asking her what had happened in the past to cause her to shut down.

She got quiet and eventually told me of an incident when she was about 5 years old and her grandmother caught her innocently admiring herself in a mirror and thinking how beautiful she looked. She was scolded and shamed for this, and as a result had stopped loving her physical being. She felt the effects to the present day. I suggested that she forgive her grandmother (who had since died), start to love herself fully as a woman and let her beauty and femininity express itself freely. (I went into more detail with these suggestions.) She stayed on the cleanse and called me on Day 10 to say that all her energy was back, that she felt very happy, and even that the lemonade drink tasted great and was totally satisfying her needs. Again, *mind helps body help mind.*

---

side effects, and still are willing to endure the treatment without question because they trust the authority who recommended it.

The mind will play tricks on us whenever our intention is not clearly stated or firmly in mind when we take up new endeavors. A study was done to see whether luck was a measurable factor in people's lives. The researchers found that the people who believed in luck had more luck than people who did not believe in luck.

Applying this information to the Master Cleanse, or to anything else in your life for that matter—whether it be a new job, a challenging adventure or a promising relationship—clearly requires that you follow one principle: "To experience the best, we must expect the best."

Date-Death by Pizza

A friend was doing the Master Cleanse. By Day 10 she had lost about a dozen pounds and was looking so good that men started approaching her for dates. She was not prepared for such a dramatic change and found it hard to deal with all the new attention. But guess what? She chose to come off the cleanse by eating…drum-roll here…*pizza!* To no one's surprise, she gained back all her weight and the attention went away. Self-defeatingly, she had set and met her own limitations.

Weight Loss

It is not unusual for men to lose up to two pounds a day while on the Master Cleanse. For women, alas, the loss is a little slower. Women tend to lose about one pound a day, but can go as high as one-and-a-half pounds a day.

Remember, it is not only fat that is burning off. Excess fluids, old waste and unhealthy tissues are also being dumped, like the junk going up the conveyor belt at a recycling center. Once you meet your ideal weight, your body—the self-regulating machine that it is—will stop losing weight.

I know this will sound unbelievable, but it's true: One woman who did the cleanse for 370 days hit 115 pounds and then stayed at that weight for hundreds of days.

Paradoxically, one friend of mine did the Master Cleanse for 28 days and found that he had *gained* eight pounds—all of it muscle! The first time I saw him after this cleanse, I could not believe how buffed and chiseled he had become. When he told me that he gained the weight and muscle during his cleanse, I felt awe. This is rare indeed, though I have known extremely thin people to gain as much as a pound in ten days.

How Long to Stay on the Cleanse

Many people will ask whether they can do a "mini-cleanse"—say, three days of cleansing, or maybe just five days. I always stress the importance of doing a minimum of ten days, for a variety of reasons. Some folks will only do five or six days of the cleanse and then stop. This is not so good. They have started a process of cleansing that initiates an action to prevent the body from getting sick. If you stop the cleanse too early, your body may take over and make you sick in its attempt to continue the process you originally started, like a boulder rolling down a slope.

The Master Cleanse is a conscious decision to remove toxicity from the body—and getting sick is an unconscious way of attempting to remove toxicity from your body.

In some rare cases, I have seen people become sick even after doing ten days of the cleanse. Such folks need more than the minimum and could likely extend their cleanse by at least another five days.

It is interesting to note that many people are so toxic that it might take them three or so days for their body to begin the cleansing process. That way they will have at least seven good days of detox, for a full ten days of cleansing. This is important, because when you have experienced the many positive changes you get from a minimum of ten days, you will be motivated to do the cleanse again—and may even make it a part of your lifestyle every few months or so. I occasionally meet people who proudly tell me they have done the Master Cleanse *once*. I ask them, "How was it?" They will say, "It was great." I then ask, "How long ago did you do it?" They say, "Oh, maybe 25 years ago." I respond with, "You must be the only person who has ever had sex once!" OK, I know that may be a racy reply, but in fact numerous people have told me that after they complete a Master Cleanse, their sex life is just plain better because they have more energy and feel more alive.

How long you stay on the cleanse is entirely up to you. The desired duration is determined by what you have done to yourself in the past, your age, your general health and sense of well-being and how willing you are to let go of your "stuff." We have many layers of stuff, like an onion, and during a cleanse we peel them away at their own pace. Some layers come off one at a time, and sometimes two or three layers will be stripped away.

A few people like to do 40 days of cleansing at a time, with three or four intervals of rest in between. Others prefer doing ten days at a time every month, for several months. Most people who are on a regular work or school schedule are happy to be able to do the full ten days in a row.

One big factor for most people is how well they are feeling while on the cleanse. If they feel all right, they may want to stay on longer, but if they don't feel so well, they may wish to come off. If you are feeling unwell, the middle of a cleanse is a bad time to stop. At that point you are at the core of a problem; it is being brought out to show its ugly head so that you can chop it off, so to speak. If you stop too soon, the ugly head will retreat, only to lurk around to pop up later as something like the flu, a cold, a headache or any number of other dis-eases.

I have talked to many people who have cleansed for 40 days in a row for religious reasons (echoing the fast of a major religious

Letting Go of Constipation

Back in the 1980s I was treating a woman in her late 20s who had been suffering from chronic constipation her whole adult life. In our consultation, she spoke of her childhood. She had become so sick from diarrhea that it was life-threatening. It took intense medical intervention to stop the diarrhea and possibly save her. Her health crisis had a deep and long-lasting effect. The constant imprinting to "not let go" or that it might not be safe to let go had come to manifest in her body as constipation. Her unconscious mind was figuratively saving her life by not eliminating. This, of course, led to chronic constipation, which she was treating daily with laxatives.

After I explained to her how the Master Cleanse worked and how to do it, she started it immediately. She did ten days of the cleanse, and did it properly, seeing me every three days or so. She called me right after coming off the cleanse to tell me, worriedly, that she was still constipated. I explained that her condition was not corrected yet and would need more cleansing. She immediately went back on the cleanse for another ten days and again she called to tell me she was still constipated after 20 days. I reiterated how she still would need more cleansing and eventually her constipation would clear up. She went back on the cleanse again, but called me once more after about ten figure). And I have known many people who have done 40 days to overcome various physical challenges that they are experiencing. The longest cleanse I know of lasted for 370 days in a row—just over one solid year; it's an impressive record, in my book! (The second longest was 256 days in a row, or over 36 weeks.)

Women Who Are Pregnant or Nursing

By now you know that the Master Cleanse program supplies enough nutrition to sustain you for at least ten days without dire consequences. But what about pregnant or nursing women? Don't they have to eat for two? No, not true. I have known even pregnant and nursing mothers to do ten or more days of the Master Cleanse. My wife nursed two children while doing the cleanse for seven days, until it became too difficult for her to manage to feed both children at the same time. (It still was impressive to me.)

In 1986 I went to California and spent a week with Stanley Burroughs, my mentor. One night as we watched the local news, a story came on regarding the nutritional requirements for preg-

---

days saying she was still constipated. It was becoming apparent that I needed to approach her problem from more than just the physical level. (I was fairly new in my practice and I could have asked about her emotional state much earlier than I was now doing.)

I had expected that the Master Cleanse and the other therapies I was using would successfully address her constipation. But I was now keenly aware that we had to go to the mental and emotional realms and dig up some stuff there. I began by asking her what she was holding onto—maybe she had to let go of something. To my surprise, she started screaming at me in anger, or fear, asking what kind of training I had in psychology, and protesting that I was not qualified to ask such questions. I was unprepared for this onslaught and made an effort to explain myself, but she stopped working with me.

Later, as fate would have it, while shopping in a local health food store I spotted this woman. I felt hesitant about speaking to her, considering our last encounter. I was still expecting her to be angry. Too late! She saw me, came over and started talking in a friendly manner. We chatted for a few minutes, then I just had to ask "Are you still constipated?" With a big smile she replied, "No!"

nant and nursing women as calculated by a study done at a university in that state. The researchers found that pregnant and nursing women do *not* have to eat for two, because their digestive systems become more efficient and extract more nutrients from their regular diets. Stanley and I just looked at each other and said, "We know that."

It is possible to do the Master Cleanse safely during pregnancy or nursing. One friend of mine did the Master Cleanse five times in a row for ten days each, for a total of 50 days, during her pregnancy (with intervals of regular eating in between, of course). Another friend did it three times for ten days each, with no ill effects whatsoever. Both women had quick labors and delivered healthy babies.

Children and the Elderly

Can children do the cleanse? How long can they stay on it? I hear this question frequently, because many children today are experiencing dis-ease from the abundance of junk food available and

---

Mom Can Do It Herself

One of my classmates spoke of a friend of hers who put both her 3-year-old and her 5-year-old children on the Master Cleanse for 21 days! I later had the pleasure of meeting this woman with her two children, shopping in a health food store. I was curious, so I started asking her questions. She explained that her youngest son had been having brain seizures and convulsions and she had exhausted the medical system trying to find answers, when there seemed to be none. Doctors simply could not find the problem, and therefore had no solution. She decided to take matters into her own hands and put the two boys onto the Master Cleanse; she did it along with them.

On Day 10 the youth authorities showed up at her door, because someone had reported her for starving her boys. She invited them in to observe her boys' health and behavior, while she explained her dilemma and her reasons for using the Master Cleanse. The authorities eventually left, satisfied that the children were both healthy and happy. I then asked how her youngest son was now, and she said that he had not had any seizures since doing the Master Cleanse. It may have been only three or four months since they all finished the cleanse.

the aggressive marketing campaigns that the advertising industry targets at them. Guidance and support should be sought when dealing with ill or very young children.

One of my fellow Vita-Flex classmates put her 4-month-old granddaughter on the Master Cleanse for ten days, with no ill effects. I know, I know—send out the authorities. But mainstream culture has some questionable thoughts on what is safe for children. Some parents feed their kids pounds of sugar and fast food every week, sometimes never even feeding them a fresh vegetable. Their children never exercise, but play video games and watch TV. To me, this is dangerous, but it is common in our society.

The oldest person whom I have witnessed doing the Master Cleanse was 94 years old. She did quite well and had almost no problems while doing it. Nevertheless, I stress the importance of monitoring elderly people while cleansing, and making sure that they follow all the necessary steps to ensure success.

Keep an Eye on Your Tongue I decided during my Stanley Burroughs training that I would cleanse until my tongue got pink. I had learned that the tongue can be a barometer to the body's toxicity, just as a weather vane tells you which way the wind is blowing. When you start cleansing, the tongue will turn white and become coated. After several days it will start to turn pink at the edges and the plaque on it will recede from the front to the back of the tongue. (You cannot simply brush your tongue pink after six days and then say you are done!)

The progress of my own tongue after 16 days made me decide to cleanse in short lengths of ten to fifteen days at a time. It took me about 100 days in the year to feel as good off the cleanse as I did while on it.

How to End the Master Cleanse

Whether you are old, young or in between, to complete the Master Cleanse you must come off the lemonade diet properly. *I cannot caution you enough on the importance of a proper end.* I have known many people to eat food too soon after a cleanse, eat too much food or the wrong kind. For some people, of course, their biggest pleasure in life is food. Ask yourself whether you live to eat or eat to live, and pay attention to your answer.

The important transition period of moving from lemonade to food will prepare your digestive system for more and more complex foods so that it does not become overwhelmed. Just as you wouldn't try running a marathon after being a couch potato for three years, you wouldn't break a cleanse by launching into full-feasting mode. You want your digestive system to get a well-deserved break so that your body can start back on the right track.

You have done ten or more days of cleansing. Please continue to treat your body with the respect it deserves. Why not give yourself a pat on the back for completing ten full days of lemonade? Now you can come off the lemonade diet in one of two ways: eating a vegetarian diet or eating a normal diet.

Vegetarian (or Vegan) Diet

Let's say that you are already a vegetarian, or perhaps even a complete vegan. To my mind, this is the best of all possible worlds for your health.

Days 1 and 2 after the diet:
Drink only freshly squeezed orange juice throughout the day. You can eat whole oranges during this period as well. Drink the juice slowly, relishing the taste. Some people might want to dilute the orange juice with water for one day, to make the transition easier.

I have dealt with probably fewer than 20 people who could not stand having orange juice after the lemonade. This is not dependent on whether or not they could drink orange juice before the Master Cleanse, just something peculiar to their system. In those cases I suggested that they eat fresh papaya, and add fresh pineapple and fresh mango for variety. These same foods make the adjustment to a regular diet easier.

In extreme cases, people coming off the cleanse could tolerate no fruit at all, and could only consume vegetable soup broth for a few days.

Day 3:

Have orange juice in the morning and eat fruit salad for lunch. I make a dressing with a bit of orange juice, pineapple chunks and papaya slices in the blender, to top the fruit salad. Enjoy fruit or (uncooked) vegetable salad in the evening.

Day 4:

You can now start your normal eating of a vegetarian or vegan diet.

Regular ("Normal") Diet

The second way to come off a cleanse is designed for those people who have not followed an optimal diet throughout their life. (Eating junk food, processed food, and animal-food products fit this so-called normal category.)

Day 1:

Drink fresh-squeezed orange juice all day. Drink several glasses of it, diluted with water if necessary.

Day 2:

Drink fresh orange juice again throughout the day. Prepare a vegetable soup in the afternoon, or whenever possible, and consume only the broth, with just a small amount of vegetables in it. Enjoy the soup for dinner. The soup is to be made from as many fresh vegetables as you can find.

In the winter, when fresh vegetables are not plentiful, I like to include a few frozen items, such as peas and corn. Do not use meat or meat stock; use dehydrated vegetable powders instead. Add spices and sea salt to taste. Do not overcook the vegetables until they are limp; you want as much good nourishment as possible.

Day 3:

Drink fresh orange juice in the morning. Have vegetable soup for lunch, this time eating all the vegetables you have added to the soup. In the evening, eat a vegetable salad with a light dressing. For the main course, eat brown rice or quinoa with steamed vegetables, which will taste like heaven.

Learn to appreciate simple meals with fewer animal proteins. Start reading cookbooks that deal with a wider variety of vegetable dishes. Expand your palate and repertoire of foods wisely.

You have finished the Master Cleanse. Good for you! Always acknowledge your successes, and take the best from all the rest.

Special Situations

Everyone wants to be special—but trust me, you are not! I have had people do a successful Master Cleanse even though they had parts of their colon removed, or had their bladder removed, or were missing their spleen, or were deaf, or blind, or given a week to live, or needed bypass surgery, or had no gall bladder or appendix, or had birth defects, or serious iatrogenic conditions, mental disorders, addictions...and on to infinity. The variety of conditions I have helped treat is truly staggering, and the successes reported back to me are even more so. If you really think you have a special situation, please just reread this book, then do the cleanse.

The most common problem I hear from people is that they are *hypoglycemic;* that is, they suffer from low blood sugar or energy crashes. This condition comes from eating too much sugar or processed foods, or (as some people believe) from feeling a lack of sweetness in life or having a "What's the use?!" attitude. I rarely see anyone these days who does not have a few hypoglycemic symptoms. People in this condition must keep their energy up by drinking several glasses of lemonade each day— maybe as many as 12 or more in total for the first three days or so—before cutting back.

Candida problems are another reason that people think they cannot do the Master Cleanse. (Refer to page 60 for more information.) Apparently, sugar causes *candida* to grow in your body. The only fuel your body burns is sugar; you must have sugar in your bloodstream or you will die. The problem with *candida* is that it creates overacidity. A compromised colon wall will then leak *candida* into the blood. We have to reduce the irritation of the lining of the colon and alkalize the body at the same time. This does not always work fast enough on the cleanse to contain *candida* growth, so some people (though not all) will experience an increase of their symptoms. To counteract this problem, they can take grapefruit seed extract or oregano essential oil in capsules. You will have to determine the number of drops per capsule for your own needs. If you take the extra steps to deal with the *candida,* you can benefit from the Master Cleanse.

People suffering from *fibromyalgia* will almost always feel worse the entire ten days, and maybe into a second cleanse as well. They will feel better when they stop the cleanse, but it's vital that they do several cleanses in a row in order to affect the fibromyalgia. Taking a product with the highest quality MSM (methylsulfonylmethane, a bioavailable and hypoallergenic form of sulfur) for two weeks before the cleanse can prevent this. If that does not work, the cause is the poor quality of the MSM.

Stanley Burroughs recommended that people on medications wean themselves off them over three to four days, then possibly go back on them, though at a reduced dosage. You will want to check this out with your doctor, in advance, to determine how best to deal with your medications after a cleanse.

Stanley gives special instructions for *insulin-dependent diabetics* in his book *Healing for the Age of Enlightenment.*

People with transplants or those taking immune-suppressant drugs cannot do the Master Cleanse, as detailed earlier in this chapter.

Repeat this mantra, please: *When in doubt, follow the instructions.*

What to Expect After the Master Cleanse

Now that you have completed the cleanse, what do you do next? Sit back and just enjoy how you're feeling now? Compare your results with the list of benefits that began this chapter, just for fun and to feel a sense of satisfaction? These are questions that people ask themselves, and for good reason.

Some folks may just want to go back to the life they led before the Master Cleanse, but I don't recommend that. That desire reminds me about a medical study that found that when subjects' heart beats became very regular and predictable, a heart attack was soon to occur. Similarly, when people's brains were monitored and their brain waves became highly regular and predictable, petit mal seizures had a greater chance of occurring.

To my way of thinking, the universe, the world and our own personal lives all exist in an ever-changing environment. If we are not changing or failing to adapt to the new circumstance in our lives, we are dying by degrees. It appears that change is not only good for us but actually necessary for staying healthy. Yet change for change's sake is not always the best thing.

After each of my own cleanses, I have found that my body feels much more attuned and sensitive to what I eat. I am no longer numb to its urging, as I had been before, and just mindlessly eating whatever was put in front of me. In the past, when I got very busy I would ignore my body's signal to eliminate, and I would find myself becoming constipated. In response to this tendency, I now immediately go to the bathroom whenever I feel the urge to have a bowel movement. I also became a vegetarian after the first time I did the Master Cleanse, and have stayed one ever since, because it simply felt better to eat differently and more healthfully.

I am sometimes amused by those people who initially tell me that they do not want to change their lifestyle, then do a Master Cleanse and quickly change their minds and tell me about it excitedly. They find that their old lifestyle no longer has the same appeal or worthiness. Truly, it is hard to go back to a lifestyle that may not ultimately be good for your health. The Master Cleanse can make this painfully obvious.

How to Eat After the Cleanse

I used to give my clients a list of rules about how they should eat after coming off the Master Cleanse. This was extremely dogmatic of me and not always the most effective way to encourage people I cared about to make positive changes. These days, I suggest to my clients that they start changing slowly—by introducing certain foods into their daily diets and leaving other ones alone. They can then make their own assessments from what they eat and how they feel and how they look afterward. This program turns out to be a far more empowering experience and produces better results than turning eating practices around 180 degrees.

I typically offer a number of basic suggestions:

—*Eat raw foods,* as much as possible. They are high in enzymes, which makes them easier to digest, assimilate and then eliminate.

—*Eat an alkaline diet,* one that is at least 80 percent alkaline forming to the body.

—*Avoid processed foods* as much as you possibly can—those containing white flour, white sugar, white rice, white vinegar and the like.

—*Go organic* whenever possible. (Many supermarket chains are expanding their product line of organic offerings.) Organic foods almost always taste better than nonorganic, and besides that they contain more nutrients and are more eco-friendly.

—*Drink plenty of pure water* throughout the day. This will help you absorb nutrients more effectively and will assist your cells in their task of dumping toxins and flushing out your system on a daily basis.

—*Beware the nightshade.* Many people feel better when they avoid plants in the nightshade family of herbs, shrubs and trees. Cayenne, of course, is an exception to this rule and is used in the lemonade. Tomatoes, potatoes, eggplant, peppers and tobacco belong in this group. (Belladonna, or medical atropine, is extracted from the "deadly nightshade" plant.)

To expand on the last item above: Foods from the nightshade family tend to exacerbate any inflammatory conditions you might have. They may also cause headaches and trigger migraines in some people. I have had clients grow angry when I tell them that they may have been sickened by eating these popular foods. I first ask them whether they love to eat these foods, and they reply "yes." I then ask whether they have specific symptoms, and again they reply in the affirmative. At that point I tell them, "so, connect the dots. You eat these foods and you have these problems, so figure it out—cause and effect."

I remind them of one more factor related to their experience of these foods. That is, I remind them to take stock in how much water they drink every day while eating foods from the nightshade family. I remind them that the more water they drink, the less noticeable their discomfort will be. I give them a simple test: Eat nothing from the nightshade family for at least two weeks; then eat from among these foods at all three meals for one day only, while paying close attention to how their body feels for the next 24 hours or so. They will have their answer, tailored to their own body's chemistry.

If you take in all the above suggestions of what to do after your cleanse, you are not exactly doing rocket science. Instead, you are using common sense and learning to become more aware of your body. You are perhaps dredging up memories of what you have done to it over the years, and you are starting to put the puzzle pieces together.

Routinely in my practice, I find that many clients come to me with maybe the borders of their life-puzzle filled in. I simply help them put the remaining pieces in place, so that they can see the big picture of their health choices. Doing this with them, rather than for them, makes it much easier to help them understand what is happening in their life and how to make the choices that work best *for them*.

Enhancing Your Results

I have amassed a number of suggestions for helping you optimize your results from the Master Cleanse and lock in mechanisms for success.

1. Read the entire *The Complete Master Cleanse* before starting your cleanse. Many people take the shortcut of reading only the basic instruction portion of the book. This means that they have not absorbed all the information offered, and therefore are ill-prepared when questions or difficulties arise.

2. Pick ten days to do the cleanse, marking them on your calendar or day-planner. Choose dates when you have little or no social engagements, and minimal travel requirements. It is too cruel to attend a dinner function and not be eating. It is even harder on the cleanse to go to the home of friends if your activities will be centered on eating or drinking alcohol. Plan activities that do not involve eating. Go on a hike, find a different community pool and go swimming, or rent a rowboat and spend a peaceful hour or two in the park. Renting movies will be easier than attending movie theatres, where people will be munching and gulping all around you. Cut back on watching TV, which can be difficult because of all the enticing food commercials.

3. Negotiate with your spouse or partner so that he or she will do the cooking and grocery shopping for the household during the entire ten days of your cleanse. Focus on yourself for a change.

4. Plan to start the cleanse on the weekend or when you have several consecutive days off work. Most people find the first few days the hardest. Choose not to do the cleanse over a holiday. It is pretty hard not to eat food while everyone else is enjoying a lovely Thanksgiving feast.

5. Line up your supporters. Think about those among your friends and family who will be most supportive of you, then arrange to spend time with them. Stay away from people who will sabotage you. Tell only those people who will support you that you are doing a cleanse. Don't listen to negative comments.

6. Gather your ingredients in advance. If possible, buy only organic lemons, limes and oranges. Ripen your fruit by letting it sit out on the counter for a few days before you use it. Buy your sea salt and herbal laxative. The salt must be sea salt, not regular salt, and not the iodized kind. All these items can be found at health food stores or in the natural section of many grocery stores.

7. If you drink coffee or caffeinated sodas, or eat chocolate or sugary foods on a daily basis, try to wean yourself away from these foods before starting the cleanse.

8. Remember that you can use herbal remedies—such as ginger for stomach upset or peppermint tea if your breath is bad. If you have an herbalist available, have a consultation about using herbal remedies while cleansing, but don't let him or her discourage you from doing the cleanse. Remember that you can drink herbal teas that don't contain caffeine, for both pleasure and variety.

9. Start a cleansing journal. Write your goals, why you are doing the cleanse, what you hope to achieve from it and who your support partner is. Keep track of what you do and how you feel. Each day, keep track of how much lemonade you drink, whether you eliminate or not and how you feel emotionally. If you run into a problem, it will be easier to figure out what the issue is when you can consult your record. At the end of your cleanse, write down your results and anything you want to try on your next cleanse.

10. Prepare yourself both mentally and emotionally. Set a date to start the cleanse and then consider what issues might come up for you. Look for solutions to those problems, and gather support to help you overcome them. Support could be in the form of information or the ability to use some adjunct therapy. It could also be in the form of someone else who has done

the Master Cleanse, a practitioner in Vita-Flex or is well versed in the work of Stanley Burroughs or other holistic healers. It could be a massage therapist or reflexologist who will support you in doing the cleanse. If you anticipate significant problems, find a practitioner early on who can help you if and when necessary, including by phone consultation, if needed. Not all alternative therapists support cleansing, mostly because they have not done it themselves and are unaware of the benefits.

11. Make sure that if you feel tired, you get lots of rest.

12. Find something inspiring to read during your cleanse. There are lots of motivating and helpful books to read that can support you in changing and healing your life. While cleansing, avoid magazines that feature tempting food ads, recipes and other "eye candy."

13. Use affirmations to promote your healing. Write your favorite ones down, and post them on your bathroom mirror. Read them aloud several times a day. Here are a few examples:

—I am willing to change.

—I find success in all my endeavors.

—It is safe for me to cleanse.

—I release the need to be ill.

—I always feel supported on my path to wellness.

—I am becoming healthier and happier day by day.

14. Wear bright-colored clothes. Spend time in the sunshine and breath in the fresh air, and out with the old.

15. Listen to inspiring music or watch edifying movies that depict positive situations, not violence.

16. Use the time that you are not spending to shop for, prepare, and cook your normal foods as an opportunity to clean up your external life. While you are doing the Master Cleanse you can tackle easy chores like primping or cleaning up your body (nails, hair, skin, calluses), tidying up your bedroom or workroom, sorting your papers and getting small tasks out of the way.

17. Consider following an exercise program. Start lightly, at first. You could begin by just walking 30 minutes a day, then working up to a longer or more vigorous walk.

18. Do yoga.

19. Meditate.

20. Use an herbal remedy during the Master Cleanse to help rid yourself of internal parasites.

21. Take a sauna and/or use a steam room to assist the detoxification process. Infrared saunas, if available in your area, are the least stressful to the heart and the most efficient type of sauna to maximize the healing process.

Avoiding Common Mistakes

At the risk of being repetitive, I have gathered the most typical mistakes that people make on a cleanse. You might use this as a checklist for what *NOT* to do:

1. Not preparing mentally for the cleanse or not reading the instructions first.

2. Not drinking adequate amounts of lemonade each day.

3. Waiting until too late in the day before drinking the first glass of lemonade. Drink it within the first several hours after you wake up.

4. Drinking more water than lemonade during the cleanse.

5. Not drinking the lemonade fresh. Or not making the drink in large quantities or in advance. ❖ *Note:* Only use a concentrate when you absolutely have to.

6. Taking the ingredients separately. Or omitting one ingredient altogether. ❖ *Tip:* The body needs the combination of ingredients to maximize cleansing.

7. Not drinking the lemonade within ten minutes of preparation.

8. Not taking the herbal laxative every night and every morning, if you choose not to do the salt water flush. ❖ *Solution:* Adjust the amount of laxative you take by steeping the laxative

tea longer or taking more capsules if you are not eliminating enough. Decrease the laxative if you are overly cramping or are eliminating way too much. Increase the amount of salt if the salt water does not pass out through the rectum when doing the internal salt water flush.

9. Worrying about being on the cleanse needlessly. ❖ *Good news:* In ten days you will neither starve nor fade away like the Cheshire cat!

10. Not using ripe lemons or limes.

11. Not using the best possible pure water.

12. Using honey or any other sweetener, except as outlined in this book or in Stanley Burroughs's books.

13. Cheating. ❖ *Tip:* Eating even small amounts of anything other than the approved ingredients will affect the success of your Master Cleanse. Do not accept so much as a forkful of dessert from your companion.

14. Stopping too soon.

15. Continuing with supplements while on the cleanse.

16. Coming off the cleanse improperly.

17. Putting cayenne in the concentrate. ❖ *Caution:* Doing so will make it "steep" and result in lemonade that is way too hot. Instead, add the cayenne to the drink as you prepare it.

PART TWO

Living a New Life After the Master Cleanse: Staying Healthy and Clear

Building on the Benefits of the Master Cleanse

Now that you have completed the full ten-day Master Cleanse, you'll definitely want to maintain those amazing results. Expanding on the Master Cleanse is easy and often not as much of a commitment, though dedication and accuracy are the keys.

Before starting on other cleanses and flushes, you'll want to decide if doing another Master Cleanse is right for you and, if so, when you should plan to do your next one. Remember that the process of cleansing usually heals your symptoms in reverse chronological order—the newest symptoms heal first and your most persistent symptoms will disappear last; this also works from outside to inside the body. Like peeling an onion, the length of the Master Cleanse will dictate how many layers of damage are removed and how efficiently your body will heal your specific health disorders. (I did 100 days in one year to accomplish my goals at that time.)

Some individuals I coach on the Master Cleanse schedule lengthy cleanses that may last between 30 and 40 days at a time with a couple months of regular diet in between. Other people choose a standard ten-day cleanse once a month for several months in a row. The way you choose to do deep cleansing should depend on your lifestyle and how disciplined you are—the right way is simply the *best* way for you. Spend some time to determine what method works best for you and set up a calendar for the next four to six months with some realistic goals. Make sure to plan around social events, special occasions and holidays to ensure successful cleanses.

Once you have established your long-term goals and plans, you can create some additional daily and weekly routines to help stay on track and continue to enhance your well-being.

Lemons and Daily Detox

Completing your Master Cleanse doesn't mean you have to cut out the amazing benefits of lemonade. A great way to maintain the detoxifying benefits of the cleanse is to continue drinking one to two glasses of lemonade in the morning to start your day. Many people report that after the Master Cleanse they no longer drink coffee, instead choosing energy-packed lemonade as an early morning alternative. Lemons are a paradoxically unique food—while they are officially acidic, they highly alkalize the body when digested. In addition, the helpful acids in lemons assist in the breakdown of various calcified substances, including kidney stones and gallstones. In general, any addition of lemon to your diet can be beneficial. A glass or two of fresh-squeezed lemon juice will most likely not be enough for breakfast, in which case I recommend a berry-filled fruit smoothie—a filling way to get essential enzymes, fiber and antioxidants.

Remember that detoxifying lemonade can also be drunk throughout the day in place of coffee, soda or a snack. This can be a great way to help those looking to continue losing weight after the Master Cleanse is over, if that is your goal.

When it comes to juice, don't just limit yourself to lemons—as long as it's fresh-squeezed without the heavy sugars and unnatural additives that are so common in store-bought brands—fruit and vegetable juices are a great way to get through the day without sugary or salty comfort snacks.

Keeping Fiber in the Diet

After the Master Cleanse, it's vital to monitor your daily fiber intake. By now you've experienced the amazing changes in your digestive process from the cleanse and maintaining a smooth, clean digestive tract is key to post-cleanse health. I suggest at least 25 to 35 grams of natural fiber per day. In addition, I find adding two teaspoons of inulin to my morning smoothie, glass of water or afternoon soup is a very valuable nutrient. A few very noticeable benefits of fiber are its ability to increase regularity, prevent many dis-eases and to suppress the appetite. Adding psyllium, flax seed, chia or selba seed are easy ways to supplement your diet with extra fiber. Psyllium, a type of seed, can be purchased in both seed and powdered form, but be wary—make sure it's organic with no color or sugar added. Flax and chia seed are a great addition to cereal or salad. Always choose whole wheat or whole grain foods and substitute brown rice for white rice in meals. In addition to grains, eating several servings of vegetables each day will ensure you're getting the recommended dose of fiber. In order to get the most benefit from your fruits and vegetables, it is best to eat them raw in their whole state and with their peels, if possible.

Mono Diets

Mono diets are as simple as their name suggests—you consume only one thing, every meal for the entire duration of the program.

One popular mono diet entails consuming only watermelon for a period of days. While I have never personally done the watermelon diet, I have met individuals who have done it with great success. One man said that he traveled as a migrant worker, picking watermelon in the south and moving north as the crop ripened. As he traveled over several weeks he ate only watermelon, and despite the physically demanding work, he reported that he felt great and found the diet to be remarkably enjoyable. Watermelon's high water content is good for cleansing and hydrating the body and will cleanse the kidneys and reduce inflammation of the intestinal tract.

Summer is a great time to try mono diets because of the abundance of fantastic fruits that are in season. I belong to an organic fruit buyer's group, which gives me access to a wide variety of fruit and vegetables. I will purchase fruit by the case and focus on eating mostly that fruit for all meals over a couple of days. Peaches are one of my favorites to mono diet with; however, they do not contain a lot of fiber so adding some additional fiber into this two-to-three-day mono diet can be beneficial. Psyllium fiber or inulin, which has been extracted from chicory root, can be mixed with water and taken twice a day to keep your eliminations regular. If you'd rather get a bit of variety while consuming only fruits, I suggest adding nectarines, apricots and blueberries as they become available.

A brown rice diet is another popular mono diet that can be followed for four-plus days. Popular among people following a macrobiotic diet, the brown rice mono diet involves eating only brown rice for every meal; it cannot be salted or flavored in any manner. This can be a bit of a challenge if you are used to eating a lot of savory or spicy foods in your day-to-day diet. The most important point with this diet is that each mouthful has to be chewed at least 40 times; this liquefies your food and will alkalize the rice for the digestive system, making it all that much simpler to assimilate.

The grape diet is also a popular mono diet that has been in use for some decades. Similar to the Master Cleanse, the grape diet is intended to cleanse the body of toxicity. Generally, you'll consume two to three pounds of grapes each day, though overeating is strongly discouraged. The skins and seeds can also be eaten, but be sure to start slowly at first. It can take your body quite a while to get used to the fiber and phytochemicals in the skins, and eating a lot of them at first might initiate your body's cleansing too quickly. When doing the grape diet, remember that you need to be drinking plenty of water to assist in the cleansing and flushing of body toxins. In addition, herbal teas can help the process along very effectively. While some practitioners recommend enemas to help with elimination, I think an herbal laxative could be used just as well.

Here are a few additional successful mono diets you might consider trying:

Grapefruits—a great choice if you'd like to focus on weight-loss as your primary goal. This mono diet is also very beneficial to the lymphatic system.

Pineapple—in addition to being delicious, pineapple has strong detoxifying properties and assists in eliminating parasites.

Avocado—is one fruit that can fully nourish your body, as well as provide essential vitamins.

IMPORTANT SIDE NOTE:
You should note that when it comes to going easy on your digestive system during mono diets, fruit is always more advisable than vegetables!

All of these programs have a common thread running through them. The continual intake of poor food choices has to be stopped and a very simple dietary regimen is adopted. This allows the body to throw off toxins without too much stress and takes a tremendous load off the digestive system. These principles are very much consistent with the Master Cleanse except they are generally of shorter duration and might be easier to do for some and could be useful as a precleanse for the Master Cleanse.

Juice Dieting

While many people call juice dieting "juice fasting," there's really no fasting involved at all. In fact, I prefer the term "juice feasting"! There are many variations of juice dieting, lasting from a three-day minimum to more than six weeks. From my experience, it is almost never recommended to use laxatives in conjunction with the juice diet, so enemas or colonics are strongly suggested instead.

Some juice diets use bentonite and psyllium fiber to regulate bowel movements. Cleansing herbs can also be taken in capsule form to help break down accumulated wastes in the digestive system. Drinking various freshly extracted juices can be tremendously useful—with weight loss and liver cleansing being just a couple of the benefits. Another plus is the wide variety of juices and flavors; this can be very appealing to those who might find the Master Cleanse to be tiresome and monotonous. As with the Master Cleanse, it is important to drink your juices quickly after preparation to ensure maximum enzyme content for best results.

A wide selection of fruits and vegetables are very important to doing a successful juice diet. Always go organic whenever possible and pick the freshest produce you can find. Always remove bruised or blemished areas and be careful to cut away any mold that may be visible. Wash well and cut into pieces that easily fit into your juicer.

Incorporating fresh juice into your regular diet can have fantastic health benefits. Fruit and vegetable juices are packed with minerals, vitamins, enzymes and phytonutrients that are readily absorbed by the body without needing much digestive energy. And for those people taking supplements, they may find fresh fruit and vegetable juices are a great alternative to hard-to-assimilate vitamins. A great habit to adopt is drinking at least one or two glasses of freshly squeezed juice every day.

As a mainstay, I like to use carrots and will add other vegetables such as celery, beets and cabbage for a wider variety of nutrients. A clove of fresh garlic or some fresh ginger root can also be added for those feeling a little bolder. Don't forget to add various greens such as spinach, arugula, watercress, parsley, kale, lettuce or other greens to any juice because of their high chlorophyll content, protein and additional nutrients.

There are literally dozens of fruits and vegetables that can be used for juicing and there are limitless combinations that can be tried. Here are just a few of my favorite combinations that I highly recommend:

- Beet, celery, spinach, parsley and ginger
- Watermelon and cantaloupe
- Strawberry, pineapple and orange
- Carrot, garlic and kale
- Cucumber, lemon, spinach and lettuce

Before you attempt a juice diet, remember that a high-quality juicer is an absolute must and you should try to find one that juices thoroughly, cleans out easily and extracts all that delicious pulp. I personally prefer using a Greenstar Juicer. The Greenstar masticates and then presses the produce through a screen—be wary though, while it works better than a centrifugal juicer, the Greenstar Juicers are considerably costlier. Take your time and find a juicer that fits your budget and that meets your needs.

Water Fasting

While I've never tried water fasting, I have treated several people who used this technique as a regular part of their health regimen; although most preferred the Master Cleanse because of simplicity and the abundance of energy that generally is experienced while using it. In strong contrast to the Master Cleanse, the majority of people that are water fasting need to keep still and are often lying down the majority of the time. This, for many people, could be much more emotionally demanding than doing a Master Cleanse. My friend Tamara went to Panama and did a three-week water fast at a retreat and found that it was much easier than she expected. However, she did not have much energy while doing it and did experience a few health problems. There also can be a several-week recovery time after the fast. During this time only fruit is eaten because it is the easiest food to digest. An exercise routine has to be adopted to regenerate the loss of muscle mass, which can be significant. One should only do water fasting with someone experienced in the therapy—water fasting, more so than the Master Cleanse, is not well understood but has been around for centuries.

Liver and Gallbladder Flushes

After completing the Master Cleanse detox, you may be interested in some additional, simple detoxifying procedures that can greatly enhance your life and health.

The largest organ contained within the body is the human liver, weighing nearly three pounds. Without it, you could not survive more than a day. This complex and hardworking organ performs over 500 unique jobs, produces over 1,000 essential enzymes and manufactures the cholesterol essential for building healthy cells and hormones. In addition, the liver filters more than one quart of blood per minute and produces bile for the digestive system which, in turn, emulsifies fats so they can be absorbed into the bloodstream. Also the body's heartiest organ, the liver can regenerate up to 75% of itself if it gets damaged or dis-eased— not a test you'd like to give it. In short, your liver deserves a lot of credit and a lot of love.

The gallbladder works in conjunction with the liver, storing bile in order to assist the digestion process. It is the accumulation of gallstones blocking bile ducts that disrupts the normal functioning of the liver. Removing these stones can dramatically enhance the health of the liver.

In Chinese medicine the liver and gallbladder are seen as the holding cell for anger. Motivational author Louise Hay states it is the seat of frustration, bitterness, condemning thoughts and primitive emotions. Doing a Master Cleanse is very effective for the cleansing the liver and gallbladder, but you can add a simple two-day cleanse to focus on the liver and gallbladder specifically.

There are many liver-gallbladder flushes that I have heard of over the years. They are mostly variations involving extra-virgin olive oil with lemon or grapefruit juice. These are then mixed in various proportions and consumed either all at once or over several evenings in smaller proportions. The following two-day flush is the one I've found to be most effective and comes highly recommend.

Directions

Take an herbal laxative the night before you start.

Day 1: Drink one gallon (four liters) or more of apple cider or freshly squeezed apple juice. Do not use apple juice that has been clarified or filtered. Consume nothing else. You cannot cheat at all, especially with anything that has fat or oil in it!

Take an herbal laxative the evening of Day 1.

Day 2: First thing in the morning, mix eight ounces of extra-virgin olive oil with the juice of two lemons or half of a grapefruit. Make sure you choose your olive oil with care. The lemon or grapefruit juice is used to mix with the olive oil to make it more palatable. You cannot drink the whole mixture at one time—doing so may make you nauseated. Instead, drink between two and three ounces at a time, waiting about five minutes between doses and repeat until you have consumed all of the mixture. This should take 20 minutes or so; you should set some time aside afterward to rest, and do not consume any food or beverages for several hours. Wait until you have had your first elimination before eating or drinking anything—this includes water.

I have used this program successfully with several people who have first done a full Master Cleanse with great success. In the past I've had the client eat for at least one week after completing their Master Cleanse before proceeding with the liver-gallbladder flush.

This information is from my own observations and from talking to other health practitioners. In the end, you'll find that are many ways to do liver-gallbladder flushes and many conflicting ideas of how and why it works.

Parasite Cleanses

When the body begins to accumulate waste in the digestive tract, and has an acidic imbalance, the stage is set for a perfect breeding ground for parasites and *candida*. Parasites are organisms that range from single-celled structures to lengthy worms measuring up to 40 feet. Parasites can be anything from yeasts and molds to fungi that infect the body and create dis-ease. The problem with these organisms is that they live in your body at the expense of your well-being and good health—consuming your ingested nutrients while excreting toxic acidic waste.

Parasites can be observed in stool samples, most clearly after you've had a colema. A colema is a therapy done on a colema board that is somewhat similar to a colonic. It is like an enema but about 20 gallons of water with herbs are flushed through the colon to kill parasites and cleanse the colon. What may appear to be just a piece of fecal material may, when broken apart, have a parasite that is completely white running through the entire length of it. Sometimes you see their little heads with tentacles, which latch onto your colon wall and suck your blood. You might think I am exaggerating and I have sometimes doubted what I was looking at, but their structure can be veiled as a strand

---

Parasite Paranoia

One of my close friends was doing the Master Cleanse and after several days of being on the cleanse, I suggested she use a parasite cleansing formula at the same time. After a few days of this, she began to feel very agitated and anxious with other symptoms that were causing her some discomfort. I was somewhat surprised, because the longer someone continues on the cleanse, the better they feel, unless they are experiencing a healing crisis—but this did not appear to be like that. She finished the Master Cleanse and continued with the parasite cleanse until she finished the first cycle. Parasite cleansing programs cycle on and off to kill the parasites in their various stages of development. When we began talking about getting started on her second round of parasite cleansing, she immediately began to feel the same anxiety and bodily discomfort she had been feeling earlier on the cleanse. She then realized that these feelings started only after she began doing the parasite cleanse. This was not unfamiliar to her as these were symptoms she had experienced in the past. She was then able to connect this discomfort with parasites that had been agitated within her body.

---

of mucus. However, once in the toilet bowl the frightening parasite can be seen. Parasites feed on highly nutritious food but can be poisoned by other foods. During the Master Cleanse, parasites are simply not provided enough beneficial nutrients to survive.

I have seen live blood samples with cells under attack by parasites that have attached themselves to the red blood cells and begun sucking out the cellular fluids. In some toilet bowls there have been whole nests of parasites entangled with other unusual life forms that I did not recognize. I have also seen intestinal parasites that are several inches long with a red streak running through their length—the blood they have been sucking from the large intestinal wall.

These organisms have a wide variety of shapes and sizes, and can infect almost any part of the body. Their long history of evolution has made them very opportunistic and difficult to eradicate. I have read that some researchers have discovered that certain parasites run whole ecosystems with their life cycles; I believe their effects are far greater than you might possibly imagine.

I have known many clients to start a parasite cleanse and after three or four days they complain that they don't like the way they feel so they want to stop. I ask them, "Is this you speaking, or the parasites?"

Parasites don't create your negative feelings or emotions, but they do exacerbate them to such a state that they become, in some cases, unmanageable. One client reported after eight days of advanced cleansing that her partner hardly recognized her; she had become so much calmer and more peaceful. Prior to this, she had spoken of her inability to control her outbursts of anger and rage.

The toxic waste parasites produce not only poison your body but also your mind, affecting mental clarity and emotional stability. You are responsible for the emotions you are choosing, but it is the parasites that can greatly exacerbate them to a degree where certain mental illnesses can be the outcome. A good personal test for problem-causing parasites is to try a parasite cleanse with a Master Cleanse and compare your emotional well-being before and after.

Parasite Cleansing

There are many different parasite formulas and kits available online or in health food stores. I tend to vary the brands I use; it's smart to have a change in the method you are using so the parasites can't adapt as easily to it.

I follow a fairly simple 50-day program. I take the herbal formula as directed for a period of ten days, then stop for another ten days—repeating this process until the 50-day cycle is through. The on-off process helps kill parasites in their various stages of development. The first ten days kill the initial parasites; however, before dying, many will leave egg sacs that will hatch after the herbal formula is discontinued. By waiting ten days and starting your second round of herbs, you can kill them in their larval stage before they can lay eggs of their own. The final ten days are simply for good measure.

On the preventive side, the most effective means is to have regular bowel movements everyday with a transit time less than 24 hours. This means that what you have eaten should be digested, assimilated and eliminated in less than 24 hours. If not, the parasite eggs that you may have been exposed to and ingested will incubate and hatch in your gut and then attach to the colon wall.

I also use encapsulated therapeutic essential oils to kill parasites; they are very effective in cleansing deep tissues that herbs may not get to. Along with the essential oils, I use Color Therapy, employing the color yellow to kill parasites. The key to great success with any of these therapies is to cleanse your body regularly and keep it in an alkaline state. Do at least one or two parasite cleanses a year to be on the safe side.

Candida

I am often contacted in regards to *candida* infections, yeast problems and the effectiveness of the Master Cleanse. Many people are concerned that the maple syrup will feed the *candida* and it will bloom. *Candida albicans* is not really a yeast, but a kind of fungus that normally lives in the intestinal tract. One job of *candida* is to make your fecal material biodegradable. *Candida* tends to remain in check when the body is in an alkaline state, but with too much acidity in the body, it can cause a host of problems from yeast infections, thrush, diarrhea and food cravings to depression and insomnia. In most cases, the Master Cleanse is great at controlling *candida*, though the combination of lemons and maple syrup can be a problem for some people. You may find you need to use an adjunct to help kill the *candida* while on the cleanse. I recommend trying grapefruit seed extract, essential oils or garlic capsules. Garlic can be purchased in capsules and taken with each glass of lemonade. Essential oils must be therapeutic grade to be safe for human consumption; clove, cinnamon, oregano and rosewood are effective on *candida* when taken internally. Asparagus and garlic are two foods that also kill *candida* and may be eaten frequently.

One side effect of killing *candida* can be overkill—when more of this yeast is dying than your body can comfortably handle. If this happens, lessen the dosage of whatever you are taking and regulate it to your body's signals.

There are a few *candida*-cleansing programs available in health food stores or on the internet, which also recommend several dietary changes for optimal success. Some of these programs are quite successful when properly followed.

Exercise to Thrive

While you may think it's a no-brainer, the unfortunate fact is that many people still resist exercise because of the amount of physical effort involved. If you fall into this category, take time and make a commitment to yourself. The trick might be to start at a pace that feels comfortable and then attempt various activities to find out what resonates with your being.

Whether you choose walking, hiking, dancing, yoga, kayaking, biking, swimming or any other activity, the improvements you'll see won't just be limited to your physical well-being but your mental and emotional well-being too.

The importance of exercise cannot be overstated, but should not be overdone as one study demonstrated. A number of people were exercising at various levels of their maximum performance. Some people exercised at 60 percent of peak physical performance, another group at 70 percent, another at 80 percent and the last group at 90 percent. It was found that the group that exercised at 70 percent had the fastest gains in strength and stamina.

I believe that one of the best exercises available is bouncing on a trampoline. It was a rage in the early to mid 1980s and it was at this time I bought a 44-square-inch mini-trampoline, which I still have today. Bouncing on a trampoline will move your lymphatic system more effectively that any other exercise. It will affect every cell in your body because the increased g-force pulls on every cell in your body. The change in direction with the acceleration caused by the springs can load as much as a three g-force on your body. This can force the cells to excrete wastes or toxins into the lymph system and then to be excreted by the body. Any degenerative dis-eases will benefit greatly from this activity. Start slowly at first only about five minutes at a time, and work up to longer exercise times of up to 20 minutes at a time.

Aerobic exercise is activity that uses and improves oxygen consumption. Aerobic means "with oxygen" so this involves the use of oxygen metabolizing glucose to create energy while exercising. Generally, at least 20 minutes of exercise is done with a warm up and cool-down period. Running is an example of aerobic exercise and, contrary to many people's beliefs, does not increase hip or knee injuries or problems. In fact, it diminishes them.

The benefits of aerobic exercise are many and include:

- Increases metabolic rate that leads to weight loss in overweight conditions
- Improves circulation and lowered blood pressure
- Strengthens and enlarges the heart and reduces resting heart rate
- Strengthens lungs and respiration
- Increases red blood cells in the body for oxygen transportation
- Improves mental and emotional states, as well as improves self-esteem
- High-impact aerobics improve bone density, helping to prevent osteoporosis
- Improves overall efficiency with many metabolic and injury-recovery processes in the body

Many people use a personal trainer to motivate and guide their routine and to monitor their progress. This is not possible for everyone, but finding an exercise buddy can be very useful. Having a friend to motivate and challenge you, and vice versa, will make your exercise more fun. I personally like to hike, sometimes with my daughter or other friends. My favorite activity is to dance. I dance at parties, concerts and sometimes on the streets to music played by local musicians. I find that dancing is an activity that keeps you in present time and can be uplifting when listening to the right music.

If you work out alone you can listen to motivating or inspirational CDs at the same time; this will make your workout program all that much more enjoyable. You can even make your own self-talk recordings and play them back on an mp3 player. Affirmation and positive self-imagery will boost your self-esteem and immune system.

Anaerobic exercise is exercise in which oxygen is not consumed in the creation of energy and the activity is only for short durations. Sprinting is an anaerobic exercise and running a marathon is an aerobic exercise. Any intense short-term exercise that exhausts muscle groups is an aerobic exercise. Weight training or strength training is anaerobic exercise as well. Generally, weights are lifted to exhaust muscles groups over very short time periods. This creates greater muscle mass and increased strength, which also boosts the resting metabolic rate. Stronger bones are another benefit of weight training caused by the increased weight loads on the skeletal system.

There are many different types of strength training and multitudes of books to give directions in how to lift weights without injury or risk to the body. Super slow movement is a method of lifting weights that I sometimes employ while working out. Changing your routine benefits the body, so don't get caught up in any one particular exercise regime. Use a stair climber for a time, then maybe use a rowing machine and then cycling. If the body is not changing or adapting to new input, it is dying.

There are many distinct and creative exercise programs that are being utilized by many individuals. Using a large inflatable ball not only strengthens and tones muscles but forces an increased sense of balance and body awareness. This is important because as people age they not only become weaker but their sense of balance diminishes, which may lead to falls. As a result, they may incur injuries that seriously compromise their health and ability to recover quickly.

Cross training is the use of both types of exercise—aerobic and anaerobic and will give a more complete balance of activity to the body. Strength, muscle tone and stamina are the direct results of exercise on the physical level, but some of the changes may be more on the mental/emotional level. As you start to look better and feel better physically, you may begin to feel better about yourself, which boosts self-esteem and confidence. Life only gets better when your body is healthier and you truly start to love life and yourself much more fully.

If you have been considering starting an exercise program and you are worried about how hard it might be, you might consider doing the Master Cleanse first. It will make the transition from inactivity to exercise all that much easier and fun. Remember to set some goals and make them attainable, and always give yourself acknowledgment when you have achieved success.

When Should I Cleanse Again?

Adopting a new lifestyle after doing your first Master Cleanse can be a challenge. Old eating and lifestyle habits, especially eating patterns, can be very difficult to modify even when they are life threatening—keep in mind that food is, after all, addictive! However, having done the Master Cleanse properly and experienced the profound benefits, such as increased energy, improved sleeping patterns, fewer aches and pains and weight loss, you may find that making those changes is easier than you first thought. The new benefits to your health will clearly outweigh the draw of old dietary bad habits.

Occasionally, you may find that it takes a second, or in very rare cases, a third cleanse before you experience all the benefits of the Master Cleanse. Make sure that you've done the Master Cleanse properly!

PART THREE

Your New Diet Plan

Introduction

You've probably found that in completing the Master Cleanse, you're much more aware of your body's needs and potential paths to greater health and well-being. This newfound, heightened consciousness is often transformative in ways that are far more life-encompassing than you may initially recognize.

One of the first things you may realize at the end of your ten-day cleanse is that cutting out unhealthy foods from your diet is of monumental importance. First thing's first—purge. Go through your cupboards and throw away all processed or refined sugars, sweetened jams, honey and syrups. Get rid of all artificial sweeteners—they have no place in a healthy lifestyle. Throw out all foods made from white flours. Cakes, cookies, crackers, almost anything that comes prepackaged in a box, bag or wrapper or can may come under this list of things to be avoided. Read all the labels. Look for trans-fats or hydrogenated oils in the ingredients list and remove them from your cupboards. Look for any preservatives, artificial flavorings/artificial colorings, MSG and or additives that are on the label. If you can't pronounce the word or have no idea what it is, chances are it is not good for your health. Make sure if the food you have has been salted it has been salted with sea salt or some other kind of unrefined salt with all of its mineral content intact. Don't overcook your food and especially never use a microwave to heat it. And, remember, stay away from genetically modified foods, irradiated foods and toxic fast food at all cost!

Make your diet transition fun; don't beat yourself up for digressions and find people with similar eating habits that you are working to bring into your life. Go at a pace that works for you. If you have a family, they may not like the changes you are making as much as you would like them to. Involve them in the process of buying, preparing and cooking of the food so that they feel more comfortable with the new changes. A question I often hear is, "What am I going to eat when I stop eating meat?" Explore the wide and varied world of fruits, vegetable and grains, of course! When you compare the number of choices with meats to fruits, vegetables and grains there really is no question which offers a wider selection. The following section outlines my simple guide to a new diet, new health and a new you!

Vegetables

The foundation of a healthy, balanced diet is simply vegetables, vegetables, vegetables. Eating cooked, but especially raw vegetables will benefit your health in many ways. This large and varied grouping of foods is our most important source of balanced nutrition. So what is it about vegetables that makes them vital to health? Almost all vegetables contain impressive amounts of minerals, vitamins, enzymes, chlorophyll, phytonutrients, fiber and alkaline salts.

Let's take a minute to break down the specific benefits of vegetables. First off, minerals and vitamins provide the cellular building blocks for healthy tissues that keep your body moving. If you don't get enough of them, the body can't repair itself or properly create new and healthy cells. This is why people suffering from conditions such as anemia have such a hard time healing, even the most minor of flesh wounds. Malnutrition does not necessarily go hand in hand with caloric starvation—even someone suffering from obesity can still be starving their body of the minerals and vitamins it needs. The fact is, too much junk food, meat, dairy and refined grains leaves the body without the nutrition it really needs.

Second is chlorophyll—the green behind the vegetable. This amazing, life-building substance is stunningly almost identical to the hemoglobin in human blood cells; the significant difference is that hemoglobin's central iron atom is replaced by magnesium. When digested, the chlorophyll in plants helps your blood deliver oxygen more effectively throughout your body and reduce its toxin levels. Leafy green vegetables like spinach, arugula, kale and collard greens are your highest source of straight chlorophyll. Make sure to eat plenty of salads and maybe even mix some leafy greens in with your fruit smoothies for an added health kick.

Vegetables are very high in enzymes, which are needed by almost every chemical reaction in the body. They are absolutely necessary for digestion and make for less stress on the digestive system when present in the food you eat. Enzymes are, however, very sensitive to heat and many are destroyed at temperatures over 118 degrees. So the more raw food consumed, the better your health will be. Enzyme depletion is a major problem with the majority of people because they consume mostly cooked and processed foods, which have no enzyme activity. Our body needs adequate enzymes to also cleanse the body of unhealthy or dead cells and to facilitate the breaking down of waste build-up in the digestive system.

Phytonutrients are immune boosting, health promoting and also act as antioxidants. They help protect the body from cancer and heart dis-ease, and their presence can sometimes be recognized by their color in foods.

Alkaline salts are the chemicals found in vegetables that help to neutralize acid build-up in the blood and tissues. This is a very important function because almost all illnesses arise from an over-acid condition of the body.

Vegetables have a high water content coupled with high fiber and low fat. This combination is ideal for our digestive system to function at its optimal level. Peristalsis is the wave-like contraction of the muscles in the alimentary canal that propels our food through the body. This absolutely crucial step can only properly occur if adequate amounts of fiber are present in the foods you eat. These indigestible proteins are bulking agents that swell to provide resistance, which the muscles can push up against. As the muscles contract, the chyme (digested food) is moved forward at a regular pace so that nutrients are absorbed in the small intestine. The chyme is then dumped into the large intestine where most of the water is absorbed. This condenses the soft waste into more solid waste. From this point it is readily moved through the rest of the colon to be eliminated by a bowel movement. Fiber also soaks up acidity like a sponge and then works like a broom to move wastes out of the body. Meat and dairy products by comparison move through your body at one-quarter of the pace of fruit and vegetables; it is no wonder that billions of dollars are spent on laxatives every year.

I make an effort to eat a wide variety of vegetables in my diet; I may however eat only one or two vegetables at a meal. I go out almost every day because of my business and this allows me to go shopping and see what has recently arrived in the produce section and I will pick what appeals to me to eat for the next few meals. It could be fresh asparagus, yellow wax beans, artichoke or a freshly cut banana squash. With my fresh vegetables I might eat quinoa or some type of whole-grain rice. I will steam some of the vegetables and will eat some raw or have a salad in which I add avocado, cucumber, tomatoes and sprouts. My friend Tamara will make salads with 12 or more items that are very tasty and nutritious and almost always different from day to day. You can be extremely creative with what you put into your salads and the way you choose to cut them up, and, of course, there is the dressing. I don't use too many bottled dressings but there are some good ones out there. Personally, I often use a very good quality of olive oil, balsamic vinegar with chipotle pepper for my salads. Gomascio is a toasted and ground sesame condiment that I also sometimes put on my salad. Some people like to use fresh lemon in their salads; I don't. This often makes people laugh—but they forget how many lemons I have eaten in my life.

I do eat various beans and lentils, sometimes in salads, soups or as main dishes but I do not eat a lot of soy beans or tofu. I have noticed that people who eat a lot of soy foods often develop digestive problems, especially those that drink soy milk from Tetra packs—packaging that allows perishable foods to be stored unrefrigerated—means the foods are stripped of nutrients. I also avoid eating a lot of the nightshade family of foods, which include tomatoes, potatoes, peppers and eggplant. It is the sweet peppers I avoid the most. I actually believe hot peppers are good for you and generally can't be overeaten because of their heat. I never eat eggplant but tomatoes and potatoes I may eat a couple times a week. The nightshade foods tend to exacerbate inflammatory conditions in the body and cause pain and headaches in others. I personally have experienced headaches from eating too many of these foods but my sensitivity has lessened over the years.

Be adventuresome and willing to try different vegetables in your day-to-day diet. Ask friends what they like to eat and get their recipes. Potlucks are a great way to get exposed to many different dishes, and people are often willing to share their recipes with you at an event of that sort. Where I live, there are open potlucks so people can experience raw and vegan dishes and sometimes hear a speaker address some pertinent issue on health or the environment. You might look in local health food stores for postings or on the internet for what may be available in your region or area.

Fruit, Smoothies and Nature's Desserts

When it comes to the most delicious way to get your nutrients, antioxidants and life-saving vitamins, look to the trees—the answer is always fruit. Every year we hear the same unfortunate fact: The average American just doesn't eat enough fruit. Of course, not every fruit is created equal, and knowing which ones will supercharge your body and which ones will overload you with sugar is vital.

Personally, I can't get enough fruit. I make a smoothie almost every day mixing a pineapple, papaya, mango with orange juice as a base and an assortment of berries, which can be fresh or frozen. I spend several days each summer picking 50 pounds or more of strawberries, raspberries and various berries grown near where I live. I will also add pomegranate juice and/or cranberry juice as well, depending on what I have available. Remember you don't have to add every fruit in every smoothie. You can mix it up for a change in flavors, but also to give the body a different mix of nutrients from day to day.

I also add a water-soluble fiber, inulin, to the smoothies with a green food powder. Some people use chlorella, spirulina or barley grass powder, to name just a few of the selections that are available in stores or online. There are now many pre-packaged powders that have protein, essential fatty acids, mixed with berries or fruit.

I cannot overstate the importance of a good blender. I use a Blendtec blender to make my smoothies and to prepare other foods for eating. Having a good blender that is powerful enough to mix, grind or liquefy almost anything is important. I have burned out a few blenders in the past, so invest in a good blender that will last many years.

I also eat fruit without any preparation other than washing or using a knife to cut it into pieces. It is best not to mix fruit with other foods to avoid improper food combining and possible digestion issues.

When watermelon (a delicious treat that can't really be considered a fruit) is in season, I will buy a whole watermelon and eat it all over a two- or three-day period. I will sometimes eat only watermelon for one or two meals of the day and also in between meals. This is described as a mono meal; only one food is eaten at a time and makes digestion very easy and efficient. When there is an abundance of one food available I find I might eat it several times because it is at its peak quality and nutritional value and throughout the rest of the year its quality and nutritional value may be significantly diminished. Our early hunter/gatherer ancestors moved from area to area gathering and picking foods that were in season and ate only that food until the supply was gone. I, for example, will start with cherries, then move on to apricots, then plums, peaches, pears and then apples as the season progresses.

Tropical fruit is generally available all year round, so blend them freely into your smoothies when they are available locally, and in season. Mangoes are the most abundant tropical fruit grown and many varieties are available throughout the year. I like to eat them fresh, dried and sometimes in my smoothies. Papaya and pineapple are two superb fruits high in digestive enzymes, which can help reduce inflammation in the body. When you add nutrient-rich bananas to your smoothies, you'll get a much smoother, thicker beverage.

The benefits of many berries cannot be overlooked. Berries are very high in antioxidants, which protect the body from free radicals. Free radicals are compounds that steal electrons from healthy cells, causing them to oxidize or degrade and become dysfunctional and burdensome to the body. Free radicals are believed to increase the risk of cancer, heart disease, Alzheimer's disease and Parkinson's disease, to name a few. Aging of the body is caused by oxidation from free radicals, which is akin to water causing rust; antioxidants can dramatically slow this process down. Blackberries, blueberries, raspberries, cranberries, strawberries, acai berries and goji berries are the highest in antioxidants. I love to eat most berries fresh and also use them in my baking. My freezer is always well stocked when the growing season is over so that I have ready access when I desire them. Remember, eat several servings of fruit and berries a day for optimal health.

Nature's Ice Cream

One of the hardest parts of the average American diet to give up is tasty desserts. One way to cut out the refined sugar and high fat of common desserts is to simply substitute fruit! Among my favorite alternatives to ice cream is frozen ripe bananas run through a juicer (only smooth juicers have this feature) and top them with chocolate and a bit of maple syrup.

Berries and other fruit can be frozen and added to the banana as well. I make sorbets with frozen ripe fruit and berries and add a bit of maple syrup, if needed, to sweeten. There are, of course, many other tropical fruits that have limited distribution and availability, but be adventuresome and try them!

Whole Grains, Seeds and Nuts

While common grains are a healthy part of any diet, and indeed often a staple, they tend to be an acid-forming food and should be consumed in moderation. I once treated a couple who suffered from ulcers. When I asked them about their diet, they explained they were both vegetarian and followed a specific diet regime that consisted up to 50% brown rice! While they thought that this was a "healthy" diet, I told them that it was probably the large quantity of brown rice that was causing the ulcers. My recommendation: Do the Master Cleanse and eat less rice and more fruit.

Many people already know that white flour and white rice are considered very poor food choices. Few people seem to realize that whole wheat flour, or any ground grain or bean that is processed, has been taken from its whole form and then ground into a meal or flour, which reduces the food's nutritional value.

White flour is sticky and constipating to our digestive system and although whole wheat flour is a better choice, it too is still constipating. If you don't quite get it, there is a simple test to more readily understand what I am saying. Mix white flour and water and you will get a white paste, mix whole wheat flour and water and you get a brown paste. Both pastes are sticky and will have negative effects on the colon. Whole wheat flour is, however, less damaging to the pancreas because the vitamins, minerals and fiber have not been removed.

There are now also a substantial number of people who are gluten intolerant. Gluten is the sticky protein found in wheat and some other grains. I believe that it may be largely due to people eating far too many wheat-based foods early in life, such as breads, cakes, cookies, wraps, pizzas and on and on. These foods, eaten over a period of time, lead to constipation and the accumulation of waste in the colon that causes inflammation of the colon wall that will manifest as leaky gut or leaky bowel syndrome. At that point, the colon can no longer process wastes properly to be eliminated normally; some of the undigested foods leak into the bloodstream and cause an allergic response.

I recently attended a conference on Celiac disease, and I was somewhat disappointed to see that the focus of many people was not on how they might discover how to maybe correct the condition but what they could substitute for wheat in order to still eat bread and cake. There were also a large number of exhibitors promoting mostly animal-based foods, which were, of course, gluten free. Swapping one poor food choice for another poor food choice will only lead to another set of symptoms and have people searching for some other magic bullet. The lesson here is to always look to underlying causes, not just short-term quick fixes.

When you do eat grains, it is best to eat them in their whole form or as close to whole as possible. I do eat pancakes on certain rare occasions but I always add cooked amaranth, oats and corn grits to make them a healthier choice for my body. I now use sprouted corn tortillas and sprouted wheat wraps for certain meals I prepare; sprouted wheat bread can generally be found in the freezer in health food stores and provides another alternative to bread. Always buy organic when possible.

Seeds and nuts are a good source of protein, essential fatty acids and minerals that are extremely important for good health. I like to eat several types of seeds, including sunflower, pumpkin, sesame, hemp and flax. I use various seeds in salads or buy as seed butters to spread on sprouted wheat bread or just like to eat a handful raw. Some people recommend soaking seeds and nuts as well to make them more readily digestible. I like to eat almonds, walnuts, cashews, Brazil nuts, hazel nuts, pecans, pine nuts, and coconut. I do not drink cow's milk but instead make my own milk from soaked almonds and shredded coconut blended with warm water and strained. I use it to make soups, desserts and sauces and to mix with powdered supplements. In the winter I like to make millet and put maple syrup and freshly ground cinnamon in addition to my coconut/almond milk; any hot cereal can be made much the same way. Many people are quite surprised how delicious the homemade milk is just on its own; I sometimes will give a taste to one of my clients so that they can experience how good it is.

Nuts and seeds are often high in fat and protein, so I generally don't eat more than a few ounces at a time. I also do not mix nuts with fruit because they are hard to digest at the same time. Nuts are considered to be a good source of protein and can be a supplement to vegetarians. Like any protein source, nuts should not be overeaten as they are more difficult to digest. Be wary of roasted and salted nuts because they have been cooked, which makes them more difficult to digest and they have more calories because of the added oil. You should watch what nuts and seeds you eat and how old they are, given that many of them are high in oil and can become rancid if not stored properly. Soaking nuts improves their digestibility and sprouting them insures that they are not stale.

Oils and Fats

Oils and fats have generally gotten a bad rap as the cause of many diseases and often blamed for the obesity problem in America. I do not believe this to be true as long as you are consuming only healthy fats and oils, ones that have not been processed to remove valuable nutrients such as Vitamin E and beta carotene. Often, the pressing of the seeds and nuts is done at very high temperature which then damages the oil, it is further processed to remove the taste and smell and then packaged in clear plastic or glass bottles which cause the oils to go rancid as they are very sensitive to light.

The best oils to use are those that are processed at low heat and packaged in bottles that are totally black or opaque to light. Buy only organic if possible and buy from reputable companies that use low temperature and package in dark bottles.

I only use extra virgin coconut oil and extra virgin olive oil to cook with. When using oil for salad dressing or consuming it raw, I use hemp seed, olive, pumpkin seed or flax seed oil. I do sometimes buy if available sesame, walnut, canola and sunflower seed oils if they are the highest quality—which are becoming more widely available.

Trans-fats or hydrogenated oils must be avoided at all costs. These unnatural oils have been chemically altered to create foods that have a long shelf life and add a specific texture to foods that people find palatable. The problem is that these oils are no longer produced in liquid form but are solidified at room temperature. The body has great difficulty in eliminating these fats without extensive cleansing.

Healthy oils contain essential fatty acids, an important nutrient for the health of body and mind. Essential fatty acids are only found in oils that are processed at low temperatures, unrefined, packaged in opaque bottles and properly stored. There are now a wide range of supplements that contain essential fatty acids from various seeds and certain fish species that can be purchased for convenience. Many people today are deficient in essential fatty acids because the majority of oil they consume is rendered useless by the processing and packaging of bad oils.

Some nutritionists recommend one to three tablespoons of flax and or hemp seed a day. I have met several people that tell me they changed their health completely including reversing skin problems, hormonal problems and weight gain by just consuming high quality oils such as flax seed, olive and hemp seed oil. Avocados are also a good source of oils and can be simply added to a salad.

I keep my flax seed oil in the freezer to prolong its shelf life, but olive oil and coconut oil I leave at room temperature. Oils are essential to your body working properly, choose healthy ones and store them properly.

Meat

If you are a lover of meat, you may find this section to be particularly hard to handle. The subject of eating meat has made for some of the most politically, emotionally charged conversations I have had with people who are trying to eat healthier.

Let's set aside animal rights arguments and vegetarian ideology for a minute and focus on a couple of facts most omnivores don't know and some falsehoods almost everyone believes.

First, let me remind you that I grew up a voracious meat eater—often consuming animal products three times a day until I did my first Master Cleanse—so I know where you're coming from. Now to the common misconceptions and cold-cut facts.

I need the protein in meat to stay healthy. One of the most common misconceptions about vegetarians is that they can't build the same amount of muscle and strength as people who have meat in their diet. This simply isn't true. My 26-year-old daughter, Adia, has been a vegetarian for her whole life. In school she participated in various sports such as soccer, football and wrestling. The sport she excelled at was wrestling. She became a national gold- and silver-medal winner and, in one tournament, beat a competitor that had placed third in the world. I would hear coaches complain that my daughter Adia would just out-muscle their athletes!

So where's the protein? I hear this question constantly when I tell people that I am either on the Master Cleanse or that I am a vegetarian. It's rather ironic to think that meat and dairy products are procured from animals that eat strictly plant-based diets but are supposedly healthier when it comes to procuring protein.

The truth is, protein is universally found in all vegetables. Eating grains, beans and nuts as part of a vegetarian diet will supply all the necessary protein to live a healthy life. There are of course, various percentages of protein content in foods and different amino acid compliments. The human body will store amino acids in a pool from which to draw upon to create proteins as the body requires them. This precludes the need to eat balanced proteins at each meal such as combining beans and rice.

The recommended daily allowance for a 150-pound person is 55 grams of protein a day, this is only two ounces. A 200-pound person requires 74 grams of protein per day (or less than three ounces). This is readily done on a vegetarian diet without the burden of animal proteins causing acid waste in the body.

Aren't humans designed to eat vegetables and meat? No. Our bodies are unlike those of carnivores; our teeth are not specifically designed for ripping flesh, nor do we have claws or beaks for hunting. We cannot run fast enough to catch most prey. We do not have the digestive tracts of a carnivore, making it clear that we were primarily made for what comes out of the earth, not what eats it. If you compare a carnivore to a human being, there are a number of critical physical differences. Our digestive system is very long and convoluted through most of its length while carnivores have a much shorter digestive system with smoother walls. The nutrients in meat do not require a long time for digestion to be released which works well for shorter digestive systems. In humans, the longer lengths and twisting walls of the intestines coupled with the zero fiber and high-fat content of meat makes it move through the digestive system at a snail's pace. This gives time for the meat to putrefy and create a toxic load that can cause colon cancer and put an extra burden on the liver. This slow pace almost assuredly allows any parasite eggs you have ingested to incubate and hatch in your colon, creating whole new communities and a wealth of new problems.

Now to some very ugly truths you may never have known about meat.

A recent medical study called for monitoring the cholesterol levels of children as young as 2 years of age. The study also suggested that children as young as 8 be put on medication for high cholesterol. This sounds preposterous. Could we possibly look at what these children are being fed first and then make more sound choices instead of getting them hooked on drugs at this very early age? This is a case of denial on such a grand scale that, by comparison, any conspiracy theory seems a minor irritation in my estimation.

The fact is that meat is directly linked to a number of health conditions, including several types of cancer and heart disease; coincidentally these are the number one and two causes of death in America.

This point was made shockingly clear when I heard a doctor speak on the subject of vegetarianism and its various health benefits. The doctor, a vegetarian himself, spoke of the events that had led him to open his mind to taking up a meat-free diet. Interning at a hospital, the doctor was scheduled to assist in an open heart bypass surgery. The hospital was short-staffed, so he was asked to go in and take several vials of blood for the lab. He extracted the blood and took the vials to the lab and stood them up to let them settle. Returning to the lab a bit later, he began to examine the vials and run tests when he noticed a thick milky substance floating on top of the blood. Stumped for a minute, he soon came to the horrific realization that the patient had *fat* floating in his blood.

The next day in the operating room he was able to see this man's heart and arteries and how much plaque had accumulated in them. After the surgery, he approached the patient and asked him what he had eaten the meal before coming to the hospital. The patient said that he had been to a fast-food restaurant and had a burger, fries and a shake as his last meal (it almost was). This was enough for this doctor to change his whole lifestyle— permanently forsaking meat and dairy products.

If the effects of fatty meats on your most vital internal engine aren't enough, let me throw out a couple more frightening facts.

In order to raise large quantities of "healthy" animals for human consumption, the meat industry uses 70 percent of the antibiotics manufactured today in animal feed. When it comes to beef, what cows are eating for dinner these days is just unnatural. Cattle used to range freely, eating mostly grasses and plants; but today most are in feed lots eating grains, corn and beans to fatten them up, with the addition of growth hormones and antibiotics. The consequences of this unnatural diet for them, of course, are passed on to the next species up the food chain: humans. And all those antibiotics and hormones? They're going right into your body as well. When you digest those hormones they do the same thing to you: they will fatten you up.

In any ecosystem, the animal at the top of the food chain always has the greatest concentration of toxicity. Meat eaters, the absolute top of the chain, experience the highest accumulation of a number of toxins. This unfortunate fact became very apparent when breast milk was compared between vegetarians and meat eaters. Evidence has shown that the breast milk from meat and fish eaters had much higher levels of pesticides, PCB's and heavy metals than vegetarian women. Women can reduce the toxic load of their breast milk by eliminating meat, fish and dairy from their diets as well as minimizing their exposure to plastics, Teflon and other harmful chemicals. Breast tissue has a high concentration of fatty tissue and will readily store toxins in this area and then release them to nursing babies.

Moral and Ethical Issues

The beef industry is riddled with animal rights violations. One of the biggest, and one particularly dangerous for humans, was the decision to start feeding cows the byproducts of other cows. Not only did the meat industry turn cows into carnivores, they had even more bizarre aspirations to make them into cannibals. There was only one small problem: This brilliant idea created mad cow disease, the horrendous disorder where proteins from consumed brainstem tissues literally devour the brain. These first infected animals were actually taken to slaughterhouses to be packaged up and sold to the unwary consumer. When these infected animals got into the food chain, they infected the humans who ate the meat and several deaths were recorded.

I grew up in a small rural community as a child where I saw animals raised on farms. I never witnessed any cruelty to these animals and therefore never questioned the ethics of eating meat. It was for health reasons that I chose to become a vegetarian. I now believe that our right in United States to slaughter more than 90,000 cattle, 270,000 pigs, 85,000 turkeys and 26 million chickens each day for food is outrageous. The abuse and cruelty these animals experience is horrific; I have watched videos on the internet that have brought tears to my eyes. One of my friends had the opportunity to go through a meat processing plant during a high school class field trip. She was so disturbed by what she saw that she became a vegetarian on the spot. I think if everyone had to do this there would be a much greater percentage of vegetarians. I know many people that just don't want to hear about it; they think they can just stick their head in the sand, but you can't just make it go away.

The animals you eat go through a frightening and torturous process so they can be made into nice little pieces of flesh for your plate. This stimulates their fight-or-flight response, which sends a flood of chemicals and hormones into their bloodstream. These compounds, more appropriately called peptides, are the molecules of emotion for that animal's experience and they are included in that piece of meat. As you ingest that steak, you are actually eating that animal's fear and powerlessness in chemical form and it will affect how you feel. I knew someone that was quite a violent person for a time in his life until he stopped eating meat; he was able to connect his own violent behavior with eating meat. This individual also had a violent upbringing, which made him more susceptible to the negative effects of eating meat.

There is a lot of information about animal rights on the internet, including some very appalling videos about what is happening in the world today. It is not just farmed animals but other species, such as sharks, that are affected as well. Millions of sharks are killed every year so that shark fin soup can be served. But the sharks aren't always killed; with their fins cut off, they are thrown back into the ocean where they sink to the floor and suffocate.

Environmental Issues

By far the most socially important reason to stop eating meat is the amount of environmental destruction the raising of consumable animals causes. To date, 70 percent of the Amazon rainforest that has been burned has been converted to pastureland for the grazing of cattle destined to become North American hamburgers. This pasture has a short life span, because it is only being fertile for a few years before the farmer must move on and burn more rainforest. It requires seven to ten times as much land to produce one pound of meat as it does to produce one pound of vegetable matter. In addition, a pound of beef requires anywhere from 2,500 pounds of water to 6,000 pounds of water, whereas one pound of wheat requires 60 pounds of water. Five million tons of animal waste is produced every day in America, fouling the air and polluting our waterways. I could go on and on with numerous statistics, but I would like to present one more statistic that I found very empowering. A University of Chicago study found that if you switch to a vegetarian diet you can shrink your carbon footprint by 1.5 tons of carbon dioxide per year—almost the equivalent of switching from driving a Hummer to a hybrid. Talk about helping to save the planet with little effort at all.

So, what should you do?

If you love meat too much to give it up cold turkey, consider eating vegetarian for one or two days during the week and then steadily move up from there to four or five days, saving that steak dinner for weekends and special occasions. Eventually, give a full vegetarian diet a shot—your body, and the planet, will thank you.

Understanding Your Body's pH Balance

The term pH stands for "potential of hydrogen," the measure of hydrogen ions in any molecular solution. The pH scale measures acidity from 1 to 14, with 1 being the highest acid concentration and 14 representing an extreme alkaline solution. In the middle, where you find simple solutions like potable water the pH is a 7, or a perfectly neutral balance.

For optimal health and function, the human body must be maintained at a pH level of 7.365, a slightly alkaline mixture. Maintaining a proper pH level is harder than you'd think, but it can be accomplished by consuming a diet that is about 75 percent alkaline forming and 25 percent acid forming.

What Foods Alkalize?

Maintaining a properly alkaline body starts with one word—raw. Raw fruits, vegetables, nuts and seeds are your best choice when it comes to watching your pH balance. Feel free to mix in some healthy grains, but be sure you know what you're eating because many grains actually increase acidity. The more raw foods that you eat the more significant benefit to your health and well being because raw foods are alive and have greater nutrient availability and a high enzyme content.

In addition to the food you eat, remember that what you're drinking also matters. Try to drink alkaline water as much as possible. It's simply the best choice to hydrate your body, and it can have a dramatic effect on your health.

Grains are a tricky issue when it comes to pH balance. The truth is, all grains except millet and quinoa are acid forming. All nuts with the exception of almonds are acid forming as well. These foods can, of course, be eaten with a primarily alkaline diet because they are not as highly acidic. The body will tolerate low-acid foods much more readily than highly acidic foods, so it is best to study the charts of acid and alkaline foods. There is a wide range of variance in the acidity/alkalinity of foods to know. The goal is to be aware of your food choices and the consequences of those actions. If we have something that is highly acidic, we have to then compensate by eating mostly alkaline foods with it.

What Foods Increase Acidity?

In addition to all animal products such as meat and dairy products, all processed foods are acidic to the body. Within this long list you'll find carbonated drinks, fruit juice, ketchup, mayonnaise, sweeteners, jams, pudding and canned fruit. Baked goods of all sorts such as cookies, cakes, breads, especially those made with white flour and white sugar are potentially highly acidic. Snack foods such as pizza, fast food, alcoholic beverages, margarine and butter should be consumed in very moderate doses. Another highly acidic beverage you need to eliminate or at least reduce in your diet is coffee—yes, coffee, the beloved drink. There are now coffee alternatives available that are very tasty and also have the benefits of alkalizing your body. Along with coffee, black tea is another beverage that's acidic to the body and must be enjoyed in small amounts. Herbal teas are a good choice because they have many positive health-enhancing benefits, as well as being quite pleasant to drink.

Changing the American Diet

One of the most surprising and unfortunate facts is that the classic American diet actually does more to acidify the body than it does to alkalize it. A little evidence? It's been proven that the epidemics of heart dis-ease and cancer are both caused in part by eating an overly acidic diet. When acidic foods are ingested they tend to leave harmful acidic waste acid that has to be neutralized by leaching alkalizing minerals from bone and tissues. This can easily lead to deficiencies and degenerative illnesses such as osteoporosis. The kidneys and lymphatic system can also become overburdened as they attempt to compensate for the heavy load of acid in the body. Kidney stones and other growths in the body are a direct outcome of acidic imbalance. Excess acids can wreak havoc on internal organs, tissues and cells throughout the body. Inflammation, infections, pain, and many other symptoms too numerous to list are the direct outcome of an overly acidic state. Skin problems such as acne, psoriasis and boils can be acid excreting through the skin. The symptoms of over acidity often start as minor conditions such as headaches, muscle aches and pains and even the common cold. These little issues are truly only the tip of the iceberg; it's the long-term corrosive property of acid that breaks down tissues and cells causing the body to age prematurely. Acid is truly the root of many common problems; keeping pH balance in check is vital!

I experienced the worst cold in my life after I quit college and was faced with the confusion about what to do with my life next. It was summer, a time I never get colds, and I had not been around someone who was sick. I attribute my illness to my emotional stress, the only real catalyst I could identify. Three-quarters of the population can carry the strep throat virus but not get sick because they do not have the internal environment that is specific to culture that bug. This is a huge sticking point for people, because they believe there are these little infectious agents just waiting to make us sick—when the truth is that you have to be sick first to catch the bug.

So, outside of the foods you eat, one way to control your body's acidity is by remaining emotionally stable. The surprising fact is that negative feelings such as hate, revenge or fear push the

> ### Toxic Shock
> Living in Ontario, Canada, I witnessed a lake that had been flooded with acid rain. I was somewhat puzzled by how this lake was very clear and you could see very deep into the water. I soon realized that I could not see anything growing in the lake because it was almost lifeless at that point. Due to the high acidity, all the helpful algae had died, leaving eerie, transparent water.

body into an acid state. Emotional clearing can be a more important step than eating an alkaline diet. This can be demonstrated by testing your saliva with pH strips when you feel in a joyous mood and compared to a pH test when you are angry or in a state of panic. Love, joy, gratitude and forgiveness are just a few of the positive emotions that have many positive effects on your health.

Water

Aside from oxygen, water is the planet's most necessary element for survival. The human body is more than two-thirds water, so it stands to reason that pure oxygenized water is the best choice for optimal health. Unfortunately, much of the water we drink tends to be chemically treated and contaminated with toxins. The contaminants may include heavy metals, pesticides, herbicides, petrochemical byproducts, fall-out from air pollution, radiation and various kinds of microorganisms from animal wastes. Even discarded pharmaceuticals find their way into our precious water supply. And what do we get when water is industrially purified? Drinking water heavy with chlorine, fluoride and other potentially harmful purifying agents.

For decades, fluoride has been added to drinking water to promote strong teeth and reduce the prevalence of cavities and tooth decay. Recent studies show little or no evidence of the dental benefits, but many adverse side effects are often denied. The levels that are added to water may often be too high for the majority of the population, which leads to the mottling or staining of children's teeth and a possible weakening of the bones of adults.

Chlorine has a long history of being used to successfully treat water in order to prevent the many illnesses caused by organisms that can be transmitted through water ingestion. Its many benefits cannot be discounted, but it is its success as a water treatment that has prevented a deeper examination of the possible effects on the human body. After all, if chlorine kills hearty microorganisms in water, what is it doing to the helpful microorganisms in our bodies?

The solution to these chemical woes is to simply treat the water coming into your home in order to provide a safer water supply for you and your whole family. The water must be filtered to remove unwanted impurities and then made alkaline for healthy consumption.

Remember, your body's pH balance should be just slightly alkaline, and unfiltered tap water, even bottled water, can be acidic—an unfortunate fact when it comes to your body.

Our world is filled with microorganisms but they are held in check by our immune system and the alkalinity of our body in a healthy state. *Candida albicans* is a fungus that lives in our body normally but in very small numbers. It makes our waste biodegradable and when we die it will make our body breakdown or decompose. It is a common problem for bodies to tip into an acidic state, and when that happens the *candida* starts multiplying within the digestive tract.

As you can well imagine, drinking alkaline water is a must for optimal health. Some people ask, "Won't the water you drink become acidified in the stomach?" The answer is simple; no, it won't. The stomach only produces acid when it is digesting certain foods and proteins. Putting alkaline water into your stomach will not make it produce the acid because there is nothing to digest. I have read testimonials about the use of alkaline water and the many health benefits it brings. Personally, I have found that I enjoy the taste and feel of alkaline water and I enjoy drinking more of it. When I first moved to a large city, I found that I tended not to drink enough water on a daily basis. I so disliked the chlorinated water that I started drinking less and less and started consuming sodas and juices that were not very good for my body. Starting to drink alkaline water has made it much easier for me to drink an adequate amount.

This, of course, leads to the question of how much we should be drinking every day. A recent medical study suggests you do not need to drink very much at all. Personally, I experience headaches when I don't drink enough water, but there are many symptoms besides this that people can experience when dehydrated, such as constipation. I believe that at least two quarts a day minimum is a healthy standard and I know many people will suggest signifi cantly more. If you exercise a lot, use a sauna or live in a hotter climate, you will need to increase your water-intake to keep your body healthy. An obvious sign is the color or darkness of your urine; if your urine is dark, it is an indication you are dehydrated and your kidneys are experiencing stress. Your urine should be light and clear enough that you could read print through it. Drink plenty of water and eat water-rich foods to stay well hydrated. It is very rare that people consume too much water unless they are intentionally doing it.

Some people drink less water because they have bladder problems and suffer incontinence or are woken several times at night to urinate. I addressed this issue in my first book. Often times, urinary problems can be in part caused by a prolapsed or fallen colon that is putting pressure on the bladder. This constant force creates the urge to urinate more frequently, and to some it will actually shrink the amount the bladder can hold comfortably. Men will experience urgency and frequency issues from an enlarged prostate. Both of these problems can be addressed by the Master Cleanse and with a technique called a prolapsed colon lift.

Many health problems can be totally reversed just by drinking an adequate amount of alkaline water. In addition, you should avoid drinking water out of plastic bottles as much as possible; harmful compounds called phthalates can leach out of the plastics into the water and disrupt the function of your endocrine system, which is in charge of properly regulating your hormone levels. Some of the bad effects of phthalates include lowered sperm counts in men along with decreased sex drive; in women, phthalates may be linked to early puberty and increased rates of breast and ovarian cancers.

If you do use bottled water, look for the pH level of the water on the label; a few brands now show this information. There are now products that you can put into water to alkalize the water. These can be useful when traveling or if you are unsure of the source of the water you are drinking.

Many people are aware of the experiments on water done by the Japanese scientist Masaru Emoto. His book *The Hidden Messages in Water* demonstrates how the quality of water can be affected by exposure to words, pictures or music. Intrigued by this link, I placed the words *love* and *gratitude* on a glass bottle that I put my drinking water into. Within a couple minutes of exposure to these words, I found that the taste of the water would change. Any number of positive words or phrases can be used to enhance the "vibration" of your drinking water and can be purchased from a few companies on the internet. Of course, the most important thing you can do for your water is to purify it. Today, you'll find a number of options when it comes to getting the best drinking water you possibly can.

Water Distillation

This method heats water to the boiling point in one chamber. The steam is then funneled through a condenser and liquid water is returned in a separate chamber. While distillation mimics a very natural process, it does not provide you the absolute best water for drinking. The distilled water is depleted of natural occurring minerals and dissolved oxygen, basically giving you "dead" water. In addition, this condensed water will have an acidic balance, another unfortunate side effect of distillation.

Reverse Osmosis

Reverse osmosis is a widely used purification system, but comes with a few problems of its own. This purification process works by pushing water through a thin water-permeable membrane which unfortunately acidifies the water making it unhealthy for consumption.

While recently visiting a friend, I poured myself a glass of water and casually asked what kind of purification system she had. It was a reverse osmosis machine. I then asked if she had read my first book and she replied, "Not all of it." I then suggested that we test the pH of her drinking water so we used a pH strip and found the balance of her reverse osmosis water was a shocking 4.5!

This, I believe, explained some of her health challenges over the years. She then purchased an ionizer to alkalize all of her drinking water as well as the water she used while doing the Master Cleanse. She later reported that using the alkalized water while doing the Master Cleanse was much easier and worked more effectively.

Bottled Water

Bottled water, which is widely available and consumed by most people, has come under much scrutiny lately. Some bottled water has been found to be simply tap water. Many bottled waters are also acid, which makes them unhealthy to consume. Another problem with bottled water is the leaching of toxic chemicals from the plastic containers into the water. Some of these compounds mimic hormones and fit into the receptor sites of cells and get stuck, causing the cell to become dysfunctional. Continued drinking of contaminated and acid water poses serious compromises to your health.

Tap Water

I do not drink tap water because of the chlorine and fluoride compounds that have been added to "enhance" health. Enough said.

Filtered Water

Good filtered water that removes all contaminants, sediments and possible organisms is an absolute must. There are, however, limitations in a filtration system; it does not address the pH of your water.

Ionized Water and Alkaline Water

Ionized water is water that has been first filtered to remove contaminants and then split into two unique streams of water. One stream will be acidic and the other alkaline. The alkaline stream can be adjusted to a desired pH level. Some models will also benefit your health by micro-clustering the water—essentially clumping the water molecules into small groupings that can be better absorbed by the body, helping it flush more toxins.

I personally prefer to use an ionizer to purify and alkalize all my drinking water at home and I also carry it with me when I am out for the day. I believe that in the near future water ionizers will become as popular as microwave ovens are now.

PART FOUR

Beyond the Master Cleanse

Eating Your Emotions

What is North America's most widely abused substance? Food. While this topic deserves its own book, I'll just touch upon the difficult and potentially deadly addiction here. In our society, food is everywhere. We celebrate it, cherish it and employ it for virtually every social function. And while food can be a fantastic part of our lives, it can easily lead to bad diet or a base for a pattern of harmful abuse. It will take some will power, but more introspection to make positive changes in this arena.

Sugar is now our most widely abused food, with the average American consuming up to 150 pounds each year. I believe the over-consumption boils down to two things. The first is a lack of sweetness in life that people feel on an emotional level, which makes them crave sugar. As children many people were conditioned like Pavlov's dog; every time they were given attention and love, they were rewarded with something sweet. Now, as adults, every time they feel a lack of love or a need to reward themselves, they unconsciously reach for something sweet to recreate that childhood experience.

The second reason people have highly sugary diets is sadly that the substance can be found in most foods sold today. A perfect example of this is the use of high-fructose corn syrup (HFCS) in so many of the foods that people love to eat. Our body has to convert fructose to glucose through the liver so that it can metabolize it to create energy. Instead, the liver converts the fructose to fat (lypogenesis), not energy, storing it for, well, later. Now add trans-fats to the many foods that people are craving and you've got a national obesity and health crisis with ravaging diseases like diabetes and heart disease. A government study in United States has projected that, if nothing changes, nearly all Americans will be overweight within 40 years.

These statistics may scare people into making different choices in how they eat for a while, hoping to get healthier, when the underlying problem is not overeating but under emoting. Yes, feeling unable to express certain feelings can cause such upset that we are using food to **stuff** these emotions back inside of ourselves. It is fear, anger, anxiety, insecurity or seeking fulfillment that are the most common triggers to overeating.

There is not enough food on the planet to make your feelings and emotions go away. Eventually, the gnawing away of some past experience or pain that just won't dissipate may suddenly break through into your conscious awareness and motivate you to step up and make a change. This is a great start to making a change but we still need to dig deeper. Doing the Master Cleanse can be very helpful, but it can also turn into a train wreck if the individual is not fully prepared. The Master Cleanse can trigger people to overeat when they feel on some level they have been starving themselves for the ten days. Or, again, people might eat to reward themselves for having been successful with the cleanse. An example is that someone may lose ten pounds on the Master Cleanse and then immediately gain 15 pounds back. You also have to prepare emotionally before coming off the cleanse so as to not sabotage your success. I also hear from people who have had success for several cleanses in a row but then they hit a wall and have problems with overeating after every cleanse they do. I don't have an easy solution to this problem. I have yet to work with this situation very extensively. I do believe that the following suggestions may help considerably, but I would like to hear from other people's experience with this challenge.

In Color Therapy, the color violet suppresses the appetite and it could be a very effective technique. Essential oils of lemon, ginger, peppermint and spearmint can also suppress the appetite.

I would highly recommend a mantra or affirmation: *I am willing to release the need to overeat.* This said aloud or thought to yourself will send a message to your unconscious mind that a new order is being reprogrammed. This may sound simplistic, but that is the beauty in it. This mantra has to be said to yourself hundreds of times a day for three or four months or longer until it becomes a part of your psyche. It will make all the other necessary steps to follow that much easier and more successful. After a few weeks, start an affirmation such as: *I eat only what creates health and beauty in my body.*

Start to recognize what triggers your eating behaviors such as time of day, TV watching, rewarding yourself, boredom, relationship problems and so on. The next step is to develop new positive activities such as exercise or dance. Face your fears one at a time and find someone who can support you in this process. Speak your truth, and dare to do something different. Don't let others intimidate you.

Addictions and Emotions

Addictions often result in substance abuse, which may include drugs or alcohol. But they may also develop into repetitive behavioral patterns such as gambling or sex. Even positive health practices can become harmful addictions if taken to the extreme. Addictions are often created in order to serve as distractions from emotional or spiritual discomfort. The discomfort may arise from some unresolved experience or trauma in childhood that was never resolved. This pain will continually gnaw away at your psyche, begging for attention until it is resolved; if it is not, it will increase its level of discomfort until you are forced to take action.

The problem of addiction starts when we choose a substance like ice cream or alcohol to sweeten life and help forget its many challenges. Sometimes addiction can be a behavior such as watching TV (which can numb the mind) or gambling (which can create many highs and lows from the winnings and losings).

The first step to resolving an addiction is to recognize that you have a problem. An addiction is any repetitive behavior or thought that brings harmful consequences to an individual—be it one's health or general well-being. When this step has been completed, a person can start a process of therapy, either through one-on-one counseling or a through a support group. I have witnessed several people overcome substance abuse by using the Master Cleanse to break the physical addiction. The cleansing of the body interrupts specific metabolic pathways inherent in the substance and significantly reduces the physical urges. The Master Cleanse actually creates space so that the underlying emotional cause can be addressed with greater ease.

My own personal addiction has been TV watching. I have used it to zone out or to avoid being present, and this, of course, suppresses an underlying emotional discomfort. A workaholic is another good example of someone being overactive to keep the mind busy and unable deal with present issues. Exercise, or any health regimen for that matter, can become compulsive, which then thwarts the health benefits that would normally come from that activity. Relationships and sex are also common triggers for unhealthy behavior. I have heard people complain about always ending up with the same kind of partner. Resolve this by being more conscious about whom you attract and more selective about who is attractive to you.

Risky behavior and extreme sports rely on fear to stimulate adrenaline production, which makes people feel more alive. Fear stimulates the fight-or-flight response, which dumps adrenaline into the bloodstream. A sudden influx of this hormone gives a body rush that can be quite pleasurable to some; but this can be just another addiction. Many people who take part in extreme activities do so because they desire that surge of adrenaline while others are escaping what is really going on in their lives. When I was skydiving in Arizona in the late 1970s I jumped with a skydiver who was aptly named Zing. He loved to skydive but also had to drink six 16-ounce Cokes a day or he said he couldn't function.

Abused substances create specific physiological and emotional changes due to how they affect the body. Alcohol abuse provides an interesting study of these changes because one psychological effect is the suppression of fear. Indeed, alcohol is often referred to as "a shot of courage." How many times have you heard people talk about things they regret doing and saying while intoxicated? They didn't care about the consequences of their actions because they were not in their right mind. Unlike those who engage in risky behavior to attain a rush brought on by fear, alcohol abusers often seek the opposite: the avoidance of fear. I like to use the essential oil of Roman chamomile with people who are feeling fearful. It was used in the early Roman days to bolster courage with the soldiers of the Roman legions. I know if I were fighting for my life on a regular basis, I would want everyone on my side at their highest potential.

Some of the physiological effects of alcohol are liver damage, and in cases of extreme abuse, cirrhosis and possible death. The liver also happens to be the seat of anger and primitive emotions in the body and anger is just another expression of being fearful. Roman chamomile, amongst its many other properties, will also help the liver detoxify. Essential oils are metabolized completely by the body within two hours of application or ingestion so there is no concern of becoming addicted or dependent to them.

Another widely abused substance is marijuana, which suppresses sadness. That is why people feel happy and high while under the influence of it. Its widespread use is somewhat indicative of how many people are not happy these days. People are worried about their jobs, the economy and whatever else might be present in their own lives that they feel little control over. They have not learned that happiness is something that is found within and is not dependent on external circumstances. Yes, there are times when events beyond our control happen, which can be upsetting and cause unhappiness. But these events too shall pass. Allowing yourself to feel and express your unhappiness will diminish the need to smoke marijuana. There are a number of essential oils that are mood elevators, such as rose, sandalwood, jasmine, orange, spearmint, peppermint, ylang ylang, sage, rosewood and lavender, plus several more. The important thing is to find the right oil that will work for the specific person and situation.

Cigarettes can suppress anger and frustration and create a kind of "smoke screen." The smoke can simply mask your true feelings of anger, fear or rejection so that you don't have to face them. Physiologically, the body goes through many changes when experiencing anger and frustration: hormonal levels rise, respiration speeds up and heart rate increases, causing blood vessels to expand. Cigarette smoking causes reduced circulation by narrowing the blood vessels (arteries). Smokers are more than ten times as likely as nonsmokers to develop peripheral vascular disease. And heart and lung disorders are just the tip of the iceberg. Various cancers, reproductive problems, osteoarthritis and even SIDS can result from smoking or second-hand smoke.

While there are various methods available to help people quit smoking, I've seen many people use the Master Cleanse very successfully. The first three days are the hardest. A simple tip is to put a small amount of clove oil on your index finger and dab it on the back of your tongue; this will temporarily stop or reduce the craving to smoke. The next step is to start looking at any possible unresolved anger or emotional issues you may have and to start expressing them in a safe way to yourself and others. I have had clients scream into a pillow or pound on a bed to release pent-up emotions. Some people like to chop wood or smash plates. Seeking out a professional therapist who can help you release your anger may be another option.

Coffee

Coffee and other beverages that contain caffeine become physically addictive within a few days of regular consumption. Fortunately, withdrawal symptoms are generally limited to annoying headaches, but don't be fooled: caffeine is like any other drug, and severe headaches can leave you in a situation like a coworker I once treated. This man never went anywhere without his coffee mug in his hand whether he was working, driving or relaxing at home. One day he complained to me about his insomnia and how it affected his life. I asked, "How many cups of coffee do you drink a day?" and he replied, "Probably 25 or more cups per day." I responded, "You wonder why you can't sleep?" He replied, "You really believe that stuff about coffee?" I laughed and said his behavior was the perfect example of over consumption and it was resulting in him only being able to sleep a few hours each night.

What is this need for coffee? What drives people to drink it? The boost of energy is only temporary and only provides temporary relief from being tired. The tiredness, I believe, is generally caused by not dealing with blocked negative emotions. These emotions, when unresolved or buried, will act like a pressure cooker and continually put pressure on the lid until it bursts or until a "pressure valve" is opened.

When I was about 12 years old, I had an experience that taught me an important life lesson, which helped me better understand tiredness. One day after our teacher had left the classroom, I was standing next to my classmate and talking about an assignment when I felt a tap on my back. When I turned to see who it was, I was kicked so hard that I fell to my knees. I got back up and returned to my desk, though I cried from extreme pain. The kick was not done as an attack necessarily but as a way to impress a girl. In my pain, I decided to hate this boy, who had been a friend and playmate. I decided that I would hate him for the rest of my life. For the next two days I had to constantly remind myself that I had to hate this former friend. That was one of the few times in my life that I experienced a constant tiredness, I immediately made the association between my hate and my tiredness. With this realization, I decided to stop hating him and my tiredness stopped.

If you drink coffee and find that you can't go through the day without it, you are probably addicted to it. It may not seem to be a very serious addiction, but the long-term consequences can be serious.

Although coffee may boost our energy levels for a time, it actually induces stress by pushing the adrenal glands to produce hormones that create the fight-or-flight response. If we are drinking coffee while driving, working at a desk or just sitting at home, there is no way to safely direct the resulting body rush of hormones and energy. Caffeine will increase blood pressure, accelerate heart rate, increase muscle tension, induce insomnia and cause blood sugar levels to swing wildly. This imbalance of stress hormones reduces the very important productions of PHEA (dehydroepiandroterone) by the adrenal gland. This hormone increases

Recovering from the Past

I received a call from someone who had read my book and was doing the Master Cleanse because he was overweight, had high blood pressure and had achieved little success with treating it. I told him that he should have success with the Master Cleanse as I had seen many people lower their blood pressure using this method. He called some days later and we talked further. Much to my surprise, he had only limited success lowering of his blood pressure, but he was losing weight. I suggested that he might invest in a color lamp to assist his body in lowering his blood pressure. He ordered a color lamp and when he received it, he went back on the Master Cleanse and used the color therapy schedule for heart and circulation problems. After completing another cleanse he called again and had still only achieved marginal effects. I was somewhat stumped and while we discussed his situation, he mentioned that he had also done chelation therapy and this had also failed to lower his blood pressure. I told him that we would have to go beyond the physical level and look into the emotional/mental realm. I quoted Louise L. Hay's book *You Can Heal Your Life*, which says that high blood longevity, maintains youthfulness and helps to manage the levels of sex hormones, including testosterone and estrogen.

In a workshop I took many years ago, I learned that coffee is a source of the heavy metal cadmium, which is also toxic to the body and affects the body's ability to assimilate both zinc and calcium.

It's obvious that coffee consumption can have many unwanted side effects. Fortunately, withdrawal often only lasts three days and withdrawal symptoms can be managed without too much pain. Before starting the Master Cleanse, I suggest that caffeine drinkers reduce their caffeine consumption 20 percent a day for five days while simultaneously taking 250 mgs. of B-5 vitamins or pantothenic acid five times daily. Commonly known as the "anti-stress vitamin," B-5 greatly assists the regulation of the adrenal glands. Most people report ease and success with this suggestion; if not, peppermint, basil and sage essential oils can be applied to the feet to help make the transition easier. When all else fails, a caffeine addict going through withdrawal can continue to drink an ounce or two of coffee to stop headaches.

---

pressure is caused by a "long standing emotional problem not solved." Many people would respond, "I don't think that is the problem," and give another excuse. He said, "High blood pressure is common throughout my family and I inherited this condition from my father." I said, "You only inherit your belief systems and lifestyle from your family; if you eat the same and deal with emotional conditions in the same way, of course you will get the same health problems. They are the people who taught you this behavior."

At this point, he suddenly awoke to what might be causing him stress. His daughter had died some years ago and he was still grieving her loss. He then went on to say that as a young man, his sister had died, causing both him and his father tremendous pain. His father expressed his pain by emotionally abusing his son—leading the man to resent his father.

This was his "a-ha" moment, when hidden streams in his life finally became clear. He now had a much clearer view of his life and could start releasing his guilt and learn to practice forgiveness toward his father and himself.

Emotional Toxins

I was treating a client one year for a number of general physical ailments and general fatigue. In our sessions, he talked at length about his mother and how much he felt irritated by her nagging and unhappiness in life. He came back to see me a year after doing his first Master Cleanse, complaining about a new condition. He started a second Master Cleanse and came in to my office twice a week for supportive Vita-Flex and colon lifts. This went on for about six weeks during which he never once mentioned his mother. Finally, I asked how she was doing. He replied with a certain amount of relief in his voice, "She's dead." I looked at him and said, "No, she's not, she's alive and well within you!" He gave me a rather frightened look and said, "How do I get rid of her?" I suggested a process that he could do at home over the next few days. This was to get a journal and write down everything his mother did that he hated, then to write down everything she did that he loved. The following week when he came in for his next appointment he was smiling and obviously in a much better state of mind. I asked "How did your writing go?" he said "I did everything you suggested and you wouldn't believe what came out of me!" "Yes I would," I said, "That is why I wanted you to do this exercise."

The emotional baggage we carry around often will express itself physically—often as pain, an illness or just general lack of physical well-being. Studies have shown that stress will shut down muscle activity in the colon, and the "fight or flight" stimulus pushes blood from internal organs to the extremities, reducing the efficacy of your digestive system—one of the classic ways constipation comes about. When you don't process and release a negative experience, or in a sense, digest and assimilate an event or feeling that may be traumatic, you become emotionally blocked. If left untreated too long, this trauma can transform into anger and resentment—the toxic waste products of the emotional body. The goal is to consistently release this waste in order to promote health in both the mind and body.

Staying off coffee after the cleanse is key. As an alternative, some people start using lemonade in the morning as their wake-up drink and report they enjoy it very much.

There are some very good coffee alternatives available on the market today. One company I recently found at a health show gave me several samples of their line of products. The California-based company is called Teeccino, and they provide many different coffee alternatives that are very satisfying to drink. I was pleasantly surprised at the flavor of some. If you are a coffee drinker, you may not be as pleased with them, but you can change your tastes or try other products that are available.

The key to recovery is to know that no addiction has any more power over you than the power you give it yourself. And though you may have failed in the past, you now have the power and opportunity to triumph. Along with supportive therapies, the Master Cleanse might be your simplest and most effective step to overcoming addiction. A parasite cleanse would also be a very important part in your recovery. Add emotional clearing and it will become easier and easier to leave your past behind you. Of course, if your addiction is food, we've got a lot more to talk about.

Emotional Clearing

On some level, most of us believe that we are more than just a body, the physical being, that carries us through the world. But it can be difficult in times of stress to remember that we are so much more, especially when the focus in our Western culture is to look at the material things we have and how much success we have created in our life. Just look at advertising and how it tries to seduce us into buying something that will make us look better, be more desirable and more hip. Unfortunately, this may be the reason many people use the Master Cleanse, they want to lose weight, look better, feel younger and this can be a great place to start. We are, however, much more complex; we are the total combination of mind (mental/emotional level), body (physical level) and spirit (spiritual level) as a whole being.

Healing on the physical level will not only reduce the pain in your body, but it will greatly improve your mental and emotional state of mind. Think of all the times you've felt physical pain. Were you able to "stop and smell the roses" or were you just blindly wanting the pain to stop? The answer is obvious; when the body is experiencing discomfort it is difficult to appreciate the beauty that your life may have all around you. Physical pain is often a catalyst for trying something like the Master Cleanse, but the unforeseen benefits more often than not have to do with your new state of mind. After a dramatic physical transformation you'll find it is so much easier to be open, loving and forgiving to those around you and you will more readily appreciate the many blessings you have in your life. It will also open you up to other possibilities and new experiences. After all, if it's that easy to make a profound change to your body, what other possibilities are out there to enhance your well-being on all levels?

I have known many people to change their lives after doing the Master Cleanse, but change doesn't have to start on the physical level.

Hate and Rage

Most people I work with harbor feelings of hate and rage to some degree. When you stay angry at someone from the past you can't be in the present moment and experience a sense of love. And by denying these feelings of rage, they have no avenue for external expression and remain stuck in the body creating conditions to alert you of its presence. When we acknowledge these feelings but then judge ourselves for having these bad thoughts we start the guilt process again. Don't judge your feelings, give them a safe avenue of expression and they will pass.

Guilt and Denial

Both guilt and denial are concepts learned early in childhood that are buried deep in the subconscious. Chances are, you've been programmed to perceive what is right and what is wrong in life. Through these systems we judge ourselves on the actions we take, often too harshly. Where denial simply shoves our past actions into a corner to fester, guilt expresses itself as mental or physical pain, such as depression, headaches, ulcers, insomnia and cancer.

Learning through Love

I was doing a private session with a client and we were discussing a number of the issues in her life at the time. I suggested that she focus more on herself and to start a process of loving herself. She quickly responded with, "Well, I love my son!"

I said, "Maybe, maybe not. Can you give me a million dollars?" She replied, "No, I can't." I then said, "Love, like money, cannot be given away unless you own it for yourself. In fact, you may be teaching your son to find love outside himself from someone like his mother. He might go from relationship to relationship looking for the love he hasn't learned to give to himself. When you love yourself fully, you become a model not just for your children, but also for the other people in your life. This can be a very powerful gift."

Acknowledging your past and then forgiving yourself for your own actions is the first step to assuaging the problems of denial and guilt.

Fear

Trusting the process of life is very important because if we allow fear to manage and run our decision-making processes, we will rarely have success.

The key to conquering fear is not to panic, there is nothing too big for us to handle, we have to think creatively and in terms of possibility. By facing our fears instead of letting them control our lives, we take the first a step to change, growth and success.

This taking of control is emotional clearing. Essentially, you cannot change the past, but you can change how you feel about it. This new perspective can propel you to look more deeply within, and to take an inventory of your life. What's truly important in your life? Your job, partner, health, the state of the planet?

Negative feelings are not to be feared but instead expressed as emotions in a manner that does not harm or threaten anyone. The question is, how do I start clearing my emotions?

While there are myriad approaches to emotional clearing, I'll try to give you a few that have worked well and can be useful. The first step is to get out of denial, examine your feelings while owning up to any anger, resentment, fear or guilt you are harboring. All of these feelings are based on thoughts that have been deeply buried in your mind and because you are the thinker, you can change your mind.

Once you know what feelings are being repressed, begin to act them out in a safe environment—scream into a pillow or beat a cushion with a rolled up magazine. Once you start releasing or emoting, the locked-up energy you may discover within yourself is quite amazing, and for some people, frightening. If you were told to not express your anger and saw harm caused by violence it might take an affirmation like: *It is safe for me to feel and express my anger.* Another successful method is to visualize the event or the person that you have feelings toward and to imagine yourself saying or doing whatever you like to transform it or the other person into something positive. It does not matter if that person is alive or dead or lives halfway around the world—you are just expressing your feelings in a safe manner without causing anyone else any emotional upset. Remember, your subconscious mind does not know the difference between what you imagine or visualize and what you really do. This gives you complete freedom to do or say anything you like to anyone you want to. It is a very powerful technique for making change.

Whenever possible I like to use essential oils to enhance this work. I have had a lot of success using essential oils. By applying essential oils on the body and inhaling the aroma, it's possible to completely shift emotional states. I was working with a client who was experiencing sadness and when I applied an oil blend to lift or elevate the mood she started to cry. She asked, "Why am I crying if you put an essential oil on me that is supposed to make me happy?" I replied simply, "You can't be happy until you let go of your sadness."

The almost immediate absorption of essential oils through the skin and into the bloodstream will bring relief momentarily. Finding the proper oil for the specific situation is absolutely necessary. The brain is also affected because some of the chemical constituents in essential oils will pass through the blood brain, barrier into the brain causing feelings and emotions to shift as well. Essential oils do not heal you but create space or opportunity for you to make change with much greater ease. It is as if the cobwebs and dust in your mind are being cleared so that a regained sense of clarity is felt. Always use therapeutic-grade essential oils for best results and safety.

Love

A lot has been written on love over the ages but it still remains a mystery to most people. I am on this journey of life to gain more understanding and to exist with a peaceful awareness. Oprah Winfrey has said that we are here on Earth to learn more about love. The teachings in A Course in Miracles explains that people are in either one of two modes; we are either extending or offering love or we are in need and therefore asking for love.

I don't profess to be a philosopher, but I would like to share some of my musings on the topic. During consultations with my clients I regularly ask, "Can you give me a million dollars?" They often give me a rather perplexed look since this question seems out of context with what we may have been talking about. I then ask the question again and ask my client to please answer truthfully. If they can give me a million dollars, I then ask for ten million dollars or an amount that is beyond their means. The point I am making is that they cannot give away what they don't own for themselves.

When I meet people who have a loving relationship with themselves, I am inspired to be more loving with myself. Individuals who have mastered self-love are kind, generous and able to create warmth and well-being with the people they are around. No, they are not saints, but they are a little more self-actualized; they are not easily upset by the many experiences that life may bring.

How do we get to this place of loving ourselves? It is quite simple. The first step is stop being critical of yourself. Drop the words woulda, coulda, shoulda. Start praising yourself with positive statements such as *I am wonderful, I am lovable* and *I love and approve of myself exactly as I am.*

Surround yourself with loving and uplifting people and praise them as well. These are very simple steps but they can have profound effects on the rest of your life.

Many clients who come to me are feeling pain or discomfort because they are angry and resentful with one or more people and they have closed off their hearts to love. There may be a very obvious reason for their anger and it may be totally justified that they never want to see or even speak to the person or people in question. It could be that the people in question are not even alive or aware of the anger directed at them. It doesn't matter who the person is or what the situation in the past was about, what is important is the story you have made up in your mind about what happened in the past. In fact, the reason that someone may have treated you poorly or even abused you may be because, on some level, you expected to be treated that way or actually treated yourself that way without recognizing it. This is not to blame you, but to empower you so that you can make different conscious decisions to change what you are expecting unconsciously.

I was reading the book *I Deserve Love* by Sondra Ray when I began to think that maybe I felt unworthy of love on many levels. The book suggests doing affirmations specific to feeling worthy of love to change our daily experiences.

It was only a matter of days after I started doing the affirmation "I deserve love," that it seemed that everyone I worked with started treating me with more respect.

Love is a force in our lives that, when not fully understood and appreciated, may appear to wreak havoc in your life. Love is not something that can be restricted or doled out in specific or limited ways. When we hold back love in one area of our life, it is like closing off a room in the home we live in. Imagine that you denied yourself access to the kitchen (hunger), or your bedroom (insomnia) or even worse your bathroom (constipation). You could not live a very comfortable existence with these kinds of circumstances.

This is what happens in our day-to-day relationships. What we hold back in one relationship will eventually spill into all our relationships until we heal the original problem. In fact, it is this continual irritation in our relationships that prods us to heal the original event, which made us shut down our heart.

To get to the love in our hearts we have to first let go of the anger, rage and resentment that we may be dragging around with us like a ball and chain. Holding onto resentment, which many people seem to be committed to, is like taking poison and expecting someone else to die. If the people in our lives are really just a mirror of ourselves in some way, then whatever we project onto them will reflect back onto us.

The way out of resentment is through forgiveness. Once we release our negative feelings about the past and all the judgments that went with it, we are free to move ahead with love.

When we are more fully able to love and forgive ourselves, we can start to love the people around us with much greater ease. I suggest you start with the books *You Can Heal Your Life* by Louise L. Hay and *A Return to Love* by Marianne Williamson.

Forgiveness

Practicing forgiveness is central to changing one's life. A good analogy for forgiveness is that of a warden releasing a prisoner from confinement, only to find that the warden himself was the prisoner.

Forgiveness begins with letting go of the negative emotions that you are holding onto caused by some trauma from the past. I meet many "spiritually" minded people who try to skip this step because they feel it is not proper or spiritual to express hate or rage. But skipping that step is like trying to drive your car when you haven't even put the key in the ignition. Some people who have experienced a lot of violence in their lives and who are frightened to allow themselves to feel extreme emotions do not want to experience the rage that so hurt them in the past. But there is no way around this; you have to go through it. You may be able to reduce your resistance to expressing strong feelings, but I feel confident that it is the expression of these feelings that gives you freedom to move on to the next step. That next step is forgiveness.

Some people refuse to forgive because they believe it condones the behavior of someone who may have done a grievous wrong to them and many others. Forgiveness is only for the person doing the forgiving; it is to break free from the chains of bondage left from past trauma. Forgiveness is like taking a heavy weight off your shoulders and moving freely through life once again.

I was once treating a client who was going through a separation and divorce, and while doing a Vita-Flex treatment I touched on certain reflex points where she was feeling sharp pains. As I pressed on one point, she looked at me and said "I'm going to kick you!" This reflex point was for the jaw, which relates to anger and revenge thoughts. I said, "It's not me you want to kick." This led to a discussion about her current situation and the anger she was feeling. She went on to say that she was going away to do a "Letting Go" workshop in California for two weeks. She returned to see me after her trip and when I was again doing a Vita-Flex treatment I asked, "What did you do at your workshop?" She described a method they used to release pent-up emotions and feelings. The method was to dress in protective clothing, get a bat and lash out in a room where everything could be beaten and smashed. She very much enjoyed this and was able to do it on two occasions during the workshop. The workshop then went on to start the practice of forgiveness. As I continued doing Vita-Flex and encountered the same sensitive reflex points from the previous treatment, I noticed they now had only about a quarter of the sensitivity. The degree of sensitivity of the reflex points is often indicative of where a problem is located and its level of severity. (This is not to diagnose; remember, I don't believe in dis-ease.) To me, a reduction in sensitivity indicates that the body is releasing toxicity in that area and that life energy or chi energy is flowing more effectively through that area.

In my experience, treating people using the Master Cleanse alone for just two weeks will not create this kind of sensitivity reduction in pressure points. This was a dramatic shift caused by letting go, expressing blocked emotions and releasing stagnant energy from the body. This allowed for a safe space where forgiveness could start to be practiced.

Forgiveness is our most important tool for healing ourselves and the planet; angry people cannot create love and peace in their world. "I forgave the bastard" will not work at any time. Forgiveness involves the complete letting go of the past; our future was not intended to be shaped by our past. By living in each moment without the interference of the past we are able to create opportunities where great things can happen, and we are open to possibility. What has helped me to forgive has been imagining what may have happened to the people who hurt me. I have found that often these people were victims themselves and they need as much or more healing than most. I have spoken to inmates in prisons and have heard their stories about childhood and cannot imagine how they were able to endure such ordeals. This has given me the gift to see that all of us have wounds that need to be healed and forgiven and that forgiveness has to start somewhere and it can start with you.

When I can help a client identify what energy is blocked in the body and where it is located, I can then bring the focus onto shifting it. They become proactive and can make choices that are better suited to create positive change in their life. I am never responsible for them getting healthier or for them becoming less healthy; it is always the client's responsibility. My only role is to advise and support them in their choices, and hopefully this will bring them to forgive and heal.

Gratitude

A client came to see me who was interested in doing a Master Cleanse and wanted my guidance to maximize her results. In our first meeting, it was apparent she was feeling a lack of excitement in her life. She thought her life didn't have enough that would bring her happiness. After completing her ten-day cleanse, she reported feeling physically better, but still acknowledged a lacking in her life. After hearing what she had to say, I suggested she travel to another part of the world to gain some insight into her own life. I told her I had recently traveled to Mexico and was moved by a lot of what I saw, and thought she might enjoy a trip there as well.

I explained that my experience in Mexico was eye-opening and life changing, that I had seen a place where people had little certainties in life and that the country lacked some of the benefits I had grown to take for granted at home in Canada—for instance, a very good education system, free health care and a public welfare system. And I told her that by experiencing these dramatic differences first hand, I had developed a new gratitude for my life and surroundings. As it turned out, she went on a trip, was moved by the whole experience and ended up realizing that her current life was a lot better than it had seemed in the past.

Gratitude is simply about appreciating what you already have in your life instead of focusing on what you lack.

In the past, I would occasionally get upset if somebody canceled an appointment with me on the day of the appointment. I found that if I got upset and let myself get distracted by the cancellation, it would invariably seem like somebody else would call and cancel their appointment as well.

Finally, I got the lesson—let it be. And guess what? Somebody would call and say, "I really need to see you today. Do you have any free time that I can come in right away?" And even if no one did call, I could enjoy that time off.

My top suggestion when it comes to changing your perception of your life is to start a gratitude journal. Spend five to ten minutes a day writing about what has made you grateful today or what makes you grateful in general. I think you'll find that if you do this in the morning, it sets a positive tone for the rest of the day. Try entries such as:

- I am grateful for having hot water to bathe and shower in.
- I am grateful for having a wonderful partner.
- I am grateful for my healthy being.
- I am grateful for all the wonderful selections of delicious and healthy foods around me.

What I like most about this process is that the more I do it, the more *things* I seem to have to be grateful for.

Another positive way to show your gratitude is to extend your prosperity to others. Find a cause that you feel connected to and give either your time or money to improve the conditions of the world around you. This will create opportunity for others to feel blessed and to experience gratitude in their lives, which will... you get the idea.

Please don't just think about doing this or talk about it; make a commitment to yourself, do it and get started. It is well worth the time.

Affirmations and Visualizations

I believe that the *world* in front of us is merely a projection of our minds, both conscious and unconscious. From an early age we learn to embrace or reject what feels right or wrong to us, so we create our own truth and our own worldly experience. The problem is, these opinions were made when we very young, when we did not always have the awareness to make choices in our best interests. The good news is that we have the rest of our lives to evaluate what we believe at our deepest levels, and we can do so by looking at what we think, create and experience at any given moment.

Recognizing our ability to change is the first step to transforming our early conditioning into a truthful present reality. Or to put it a little simpler—don't blame the TV for the unpleasant program; change the channel.

Change begins with awareness. First you have to know you are unhappy so that you can decide you want something to be different. You can think about the possibilities of what you might want to have in your life.

The unconscious mind does not know the difference between what you imagine and what you do. Visualization, or the process of imagining, can be a means to impress on our subconscious a new or different perception of life experience. The body takes all of its cues from what the mind perceives; if you imagine biting into a lemon, your mouth will salivate. The understanding of this simple physiological dynamic can be utilized to bring a new experience into your body. You can easily reprogram a belief system that was set in motion by some past experience by simply visualizing something different. You might be frightened by dogs because of an early childhood experience; but by using visualization, you can imprint yourself with a safe experience of dogs that, over time, can change the way you feel. You may even be able to heal to the point where the fear disappears. The body will respond to how it has been programmed. This may seem rather simplistic, but many world-class athletes use visualization to imagine winning at their sport to enhance their chances.

When I went skydiving in groups, we would practice our formations on the grounds, and our practices were appropriately called dirt dives. This was to maximize our relatively short free-fall time so that we would know our positions and the various maneuvers necessary to get the most done. It really just makes sense: *Plan for the best to experience the best.* While positive visualization does not ensure success, it clearly enhances the chances of success.

Similar to visualizations, affirmations are positive statements that are repeated aloud or internally to bring about a different experience than we're used to. One of my favorite affirmations is, "Everything is working in divine right order." After doing this affirmation daily, I found remarkable changes in the world around me. It also helps me to accept what I am experiencing in the moment and trust that it will all unfold for my highest good. It is a very powerful but simple tool that I would recommend to anyone.

I have read that the average person thinks some 40 to 50 thousand thoughts each day—each with their own positive or negative reinforcement.

Here is an example of how affirmations helped me to change an old negative belief into something positive. I often would feel a sense of worry or impending doom when things were going quite well in my life. The better life was, the more I sensed that something might go wrong. Then suddenly, the bubble would pop as if on cue. It started to become more and more apparent that I was running a program that had become a part of my life experience. The more I thought about it, the more I wanted to find the root of this belief, until one day I finally got my wish. I was talking with my father as we traveled through the U.S. and I said, "Hasn't the weather been great these last four days?" My father replied, "Yes, but it can't last long." I had an immediate *a-ha* moment. This is where that devilish little thought comes from, and I have the power to can change it! My affirmation became, *When things are going well, they quickly become even better!*

There will be many situations when it is just as important to erase the old thought as it is to replace it with a new one. You have to let go of your thoughts of poverty before new thoughts of prosperity can have a truly fulfilling energy in your life. Don't buy a new couch and expect to place it on top of the old one—you won't be happy. Give away the old and make room for the new.

How much time do we waste on thinking about trivial or unimportant things in our lives? When we are wishing for something or saying, "I'm going to do this and I'm going to do that" we are just creating a bunch of dangling, unfinished thoughts that are always waiting to be fulfilled in our unconscious mind. This takes up unnecessary energy and space in your life; so use your mind in a creative fashion, which will bring positive ramifications.

Spend quality time each day thinking, writing and visualizing about some aspect of your life and perhaps maybe the world in general that you would like to see healthier, happier and more peaceful. And above all, dare to dream.

Meditation

Meditation is a practice often misinterpreted as an act belonging solely to Eastern religious practices. In reality, it is not unique to any spiritual practice, but is utilized by many different religious groups. Meditation is an age-old practice that has been largely ignored in our busy Western lifestyle, which is often more focused on looking good than feeling good.

Meditation can be as simple as taking quiet time for self-contemplation, turning your focus inward so that you might explore a deeper awareness. It can involve different disciplines to free your mind of thoughts, to examine your thoughts or to feel a stronger connection to spirit. People that maintain a constant busyness in their lives don't take time to experience life in the moment. Constantly moving and working is a form of stress that can lead to many negative consequences such as high blood pressure, ulcers and headaches. When we take time to smell the flowers, we can appreciate the moment for what it is. This sounds very new age, but I too make myself so busy I forget to just enjoy the moment I am in. When I come back to the present moment, a sense of peace settles in and I realize that nothing else really matters. I have met with too many clients who spend time making up a story in their mind about something that might happen or might never happen. But fretting about it does not ensure the outcome of any event and instead keeps you from enjoying life as it is right now.

Meditation is used to bring one back to a balanced way of life. Start by finding a quiet and comfortable place where you are unlikely to be disturbed. Sit or lie down while closing your eyes and breathe through your nose. Focus on your breath, visualizing it move as a wheel going around instead of a piston going up and down. Some people may use a mantra to keep focused such as the words "peace" or "joy. " Spending even ten minutes twice a day, morning and evening, can lead you to a profound new sense of calm. Of course, there are many ways to meditate and there are classes that you can attend to develop a discipline. Find what works for you and incorporate it as a daily ritual. Another good place to start is the book *A New Earth* by Eckhart Tolle, which can help you learn to start finding the joy in the present.

Work

This chapter may at first seem like an unusual topic for a book about the Master Cleanse, but cleansing your life is very similar to cleansing your body. Most people spend 40 hours or more each week at their place of business. That is almost a quarter of a human life! How many people do you know who truly enjoy their jobs and look forward to their work? Many people are at their jobs only because it is a means to pay their bills and hopefully live an adequate lifestyle. But what about trying to create and attract something more suitable that is also rewarding and fulfilling?

One of my friends, Anna Maya, was demonstrating the use of essential oils to an audience in very practical ways. She asked the audience members to raise their hands if they were in pain. One attendee raised his arm and said he had a headache. Anna Maya asked him to come up to the front so that she might demonstrate the simple application and effectiveness of essential oils. Anna Maya tried peppermint, which in many cases can alleviate headaches, but in this case it did not work. She then applied a blend that was specific to pain, but once again the man felt no relief. Anna Maya sat with this for a minute and asked the gentleman, "Do you like your job?" He replied, "No, I hate it." She then took out a blend of essential oil called Joy and applied it on his skin and within seconds his pain went away.

How You Can Change

My daughter Adia was visiting me one day after work and we were discussing her present job. She was not happy at her job and was looking to find another place to work. She had recently done a job interview at another company only to learn that they had put a hiring freeze in place as a result of decreasing sales. I told her that another opportunity was on its way and that it would be a better position. I asked her to write down a list of the things she would like to have at her new place of employment. It was only a matter of weeks before she heard of another job posting. It so happened she had worked as an outside contractor for this business in the past and it was a place that she really wanted to work. She applied for the job and was interviewed, and on the same day was offered the position. It was some weeks later when we were talking about this that she remembered her list of wants for her new job. Everything on her list was there.

I am very fortunate to have spent a day with Dorothy MacLean, one of the co-founders of Findhorn, an alternative community in northern Scotland. She talked about a wide range of topics, including her own issues with work. She did not like working in an office and had a lot of stress about being pushed into this position, but felt she had to do it. In order to make daily office life more inviting, she decided that she would start by liking something in the office. It turned out to be the color of the paint on the walls. From this small movement toward acceptance grew a love and loyalty to the place, so much so that when it was time to leave many years later, she did not want to go.

We have to first start connecting our thoughts and feelings to our experiences. Listen to your thoughts and the words you express. Do you use the phrases, "I hate this...," "I wish...," "I'm trying to..." or "One day I'll get...?" These phrases are all disempowering; they cannot change what you are experiencing, and in fact, they will be like leg irons to your present state. Instead, think of positive possibilities and remind yourself of them periodically throughout the day. This will open your mind to the world in a different way and help you recognize opportunities that may have been overlooked.

One day I was visiting a friend who worked for social services and she told me about her new assignment to help unemployed people find work. She said that she had been interviewing people to assess what she might have to teach in her seminar. She soon learned that many of these unemployed people had never thought about the kind of work they wanted to do. She then asked them to go home and write down what it was they wanted to do for a living. A surprising thing happened—several people didn't return for reassessment because they found work on their own.

Writing down what you want and holding a space of possibility are good first steps, but be sure to also learn the lessons your present job has taught you. I found I didn't like working for other people very much and I would have conflict with whoever was in authority. Upon reflection, I realized it wasn't that I just didn't get along with any authority figure, it was that authority figures were representative of my unresolved issues with my father. Unresolved family conflict can often reveal itself in some form through the people you work with; take time to reflect on your work environment and your relationships with coworkers.

We are always given opportunity to grow, change and heal if we are present enough to see the bigger picture. Allow yourself to clear your unresolved issues or wherever you go, you will take your emotional baggage with you. All the baggage you have not dumped from your psyche follows you everywhere.

In grade school and college I excelled in math and science but struggled with English classes, especially with writing essays. After reading the first essay I wrote for my English professor, he gave it back to me and said he was starting another class that I would also be taking to learn how to write better. Along with enrolling in that class, I also had to rewrite the essay two more times. It was like torture for me, but in the end, I got a good grade.

Body Care

You are surrounded by chemicals every day of your life. Found in your food, water, clothing, bedding, toothpaste, skin care and hair care products, many of these chemicals can permeate your skin, enter the bloodstream and cause myriad health problems as they accumulate in organs and tissues. And while it's now virtually impossible to be without chemical exposure, there are steps you can take to detoxify your body and reduce unnecessary exposure to harmful chemicals. The following are a few important suggestions you can start with today.

Filtering Your Bath and Shower Water

Drinking filtered water does not always prevent high exposure to chlorine and dozens of other chemicals—the water you bathe and shower in is a chemical soup. The harmful chemicals running through city pipes can vaporize easily in steam, only to be inhaled by an unsuspecting person during an inviting hot shower. In fact, a hot shower can expose you to 50 times the amount of chemicals found in a glass of tap water. If you're a homeowner, one solution to reduce your exposure is to have your water supply filtered as it enters your house. While these filters tend to be a costly option, it's well worth the initial investment. If you rent your home, the simple, inexpensive solution is to add a carbon filter to your showerhead. The difference can be felt all over your body. If you cannot filter your bath water, try adding bentonite clay to the water—it absorbs and neutralizes the chlorine content.

Skin Care Products

Your skin, your body's largest organ, is designed to protect you from invasive organisms and it does so partly though regulating body temperature and detoxifying the body through sweating. Resilient as it is, however, this amazing organ still struggles against the thousands of chemicals found in everyday life.

New studies are even suggesting that suntan lotions may be hazardous to your skin—not too surprising, given their heavy chemical compositions. Antiperspirants, just as the name suggests, interfere with one of the body's most natural and necessary functions for proper health. Avoid them at all costs, along with most deodorants. Instead, look to use safe alternatives from a health food store. If you eat well and cleanse regularly, your body odor decreases dramatically, a benefit many people have noticed with the Master Cleanse.

Shampoos are almost always laden with various foaming agents such as sodium lauryl sulfate or similar compounds synthesized from coconut oils. This additive can also be found in toothpastes, soaps and some mouth rinses. Some studies have found these compounds to be irritants to the skin or worse. There are many products now available without these foaming agents. Soaps and bath gels need to be scrutinized because they may contain synthetic fragrances and artificial colors that have very safe, natural-sounding names, including essential oils and natural dyes.

Know What You're Using

Read all the labels of everything you eat, drink, put on your body or inhale. Unless you start shopping selectively, you will be surprised by the many chemical compounds that are so carelessly used in almost everything you purchase. There are now many websites catering specifically to the concerns of people who have become savvy to this sad reality.

Clothing

Buying organic cotton not only benefits your health but the health of the planet as well. Why? Almost a quarter of all insecticides used worldwide are sprayed on commercially grown cotton. These pesticides can leach out of the cotton and into your body through your skin. On the environmental side, add pesticides to extreme amounts of fertilizer and destructive irrigation and you've got a recipe for ecological disaster. There are increasing numbers of fabric options that are 100 percent organic; the list includes cotton, hemp, silk, linen, bamboo and tencel.

Avoid wearing clothes made from synthetics as much as possible and always read the labels when buying your clothes so you know what fibers are being used. Various synthetic compounds are used to make different fibers such as nylon, acrylic and polyester, which are sprayed with formaldehyde finishes that can outgas as they are worn next to your body. Synthetics also tend to block the skin's ability to breathe, and some trap perspiration against the skin. This diminishes the effectiveness of the skin's ability to release water and other wastes from the body.

Air Fresheners and Cleaning Products

Air fresheners are a big no-no. While they may be pleasing to the nose, none of their smells have any natural compounds in them. A cold-air diffuser is the best solution to clean the air, only using therapeutic grade essential oils, of course. Paraffin candles are best avoided as they also pollute the air you breathe and often have dyes and fragrances that are toxic to you as well; beeswax candles are your best choice for candles.

Cleaning products are laden with synthetic dyes, synthetic fragrances and any number of toxic chemical compounds dangerous to your health and the environment. Every day more than 32 million pounds of toxic cleaning products are dumped down American drains.

These are just a few of the areas in your life where change can be made without much effort or pain.

Space Clearing

Space clearing is as simple as it sounds—you go through your entire living space and assess the benefits of the stuff you keep with you. If you live in a cluttered house, it is often an indication that you have a lot of emotional and mental clutter, which translates to congestion in the body that may lead to health problems.

I have been in houses that may appear neat and tidy from a first glance, but may actually have drawers and closets completely packed with things. But even the burden of just knowing you have clutter can really drag you down emotionally. Like trying to operate your computer with forty applications open, the clutter simply slows down your life.

The solution is to let go or get rid of anything that is no longer useful to you—a perfect personal cleanse to do in conjunction with your Master Cleanse! When we can connect to our body and truly experience the wonder that it is and feel the aliveness and the joy we deserve in this life, we will then start to connect more fully to the rest of our world. They way we are within will translate to our experience of our world outside.

Cleaning your personal space can be quite an adventure as you examine what is taking up precious room in your life. As you clean, remember, you are beginning to remove those objects and emotions that are no longer useful in your life. The objects around you have energy—perhaps linked to the past—and this energy can affect how you feel and live. Keeping a number of objects that make you remember some specific experience from your past will only block your experience of the present moment. To move forward in life we must let go of the past, and that includes getting rid of some of the physical things from the past. By physically opening a space for new things to come into you life, you might allow for change to occur on different levels.

A good idea is to enlist a friend or a couple of friends (or hire a professional) who will help you release the old and unneeded items. I strongly urge you not to do this intense process alone; it can be far more difficult than you imagine. Start with one room and go through every drawer and closet and keep only what you use on a regular basis. All items in your home will need to be included in this task. Discipline is a must! You're sure to find that any number of excuses will come up to try to sabotage your efforts.

The process of letting go can be very profound and liberating. You will feel lighter, invigorated and free; it will create space for new energy and new experiences to fill the space that has been opened.

Use these affirmations as you go: *I release the old to make way for the new, I release the past with love* and *I open myself to something greater.*

Afterword

If I have succeeded, this book has helped you usher in a new chapter of greater health for your life. Of course, there are many other areas to explore in order to improve your overall health and well-being. Stanley Burroughs did not rely on the Master Cleanse alone, but supported it with other healing techniques such as Vita-Flex, Color Therapy and occasional colon lifts. There is a plethora of massage and body-work techniques, healing methods, and emotional clearing and spiritual practices to explore. Your further exploration not only benefits your life, but improves the lives of everyone around you. These techniques can even be a benefit to your greater environment. By taking care of ourselves and using preventative measures, we can reduce our health care costs, making good health an affordable concept. Personally, by taking responsibility for my own health, I have avoided medical treatment for 29 years. Change begins within you. Be an example. In these challenging times, if you are courageous enough to make a personal revolution by empowering yourself and taking your health into your own hands, you have the power to become part of a larger revolution toward a healthier society and cleaner planet. Above all, enjoy life; you deserve it.

Appendix

Resources

Changing Your Diet

There are many good websites available to help you transition to a new diet. *Vegetarian Times* is a well-established magazine all about vegetarianism (www.vegetariantimes.com). The website is a valuable resource and is full of diet information and superb recipes.

Another site, www.goveg.com, is an excellent source for great-tasting vegan and vegetarian recipes as well as general information on vegan and vegetarian living.

Raw food enthusiast Nomi Shannon has a great website, www.rawgourmet.com, where she discusses improving your diet with raw food; she provides excellent nutritional advice. The site also covers products that will help you make positive changes in your life such as Blendtec blenders and other appliances like juicers and dehydrators.

Juicers

Having a good juicer is a must. Do your research and try out the juicer you'd like before you purchase it. Greenstar, my favorite juicer brand, can be found online at www.greenstar.com. The site contains product information, recipes and a forum for questions.

Blenders

The best, heavy-duty juicers are made by Blendtec and Vita-Mix. A quality blender is an excellent investment as it's quite easy to burn out a regular blender making smoothies. Both of these models are dependable and are well worth their extra cost. Blendtec's website, www.blendtec.com, explains the features of their blenders, has a recipe section and a video section with demonstrations showing how strong the blenders are. Vita-Mix blenders are showcased on their website, www.vitamix.com. If you find the cost of these high-end blenders to be too much, try buying one second hand—they are very durable.

Coffee Alternatives

Decreasing your caffeine intake is a must to improving your health.

Teeccino Organic May Caffe is a delicious caffeine-free blend of organic herbs, grains and nuts, roasted and ground to brew and taste just like coffee. It's available online at www.teeccino.com.

Supplements

If you choose to use supplements to boost your nutritional intake, make sure you research both the type of nutrients and source of supplements you choose. I prefer New Chapter supplements, which can be purchased in many health food stores or online. Many people like to add to their vegetable intake with a green supplement; again, you need to look at the contents and how they are manufactured. One good green supplement is Vitamineral Green by Healthforce Nutritionals (www.healthforce.com).

Changing Your Life

There are many good websites available today to assist you in changing your daily health routines and to answer your nutrition, exercise and environmental concerns. Two excellent sites are www.lime.com and www.renegadehealth.com. Both of these sites provide excellent information as well as daily newsletters and streaming videos.

Parasites

Hulda Clarke has created several protocols and devices, including "The Zapper," for the elimination of parasites. For more information, visit her website, www.drclarke.net. Other websites selling similar products include: www.clarkzapper.com, www.toolsforhealing.com and www.bestzapper.com.

Advanced Cleansing

Tamara Olson, a cleansing specialist I trained in the work of Stanley Burroughs, provides advanced cleansing opportunities, including the ten-day Quantum Leap Cleanse. The program combines the Master Cleanse with a host of other treatments, including Vita-Flex, colon hydrotherapy and Color Therapy. Tamara also provides individual coaching on cleansing, lifestyle changes and raw food diets. For more information, visit her website, www.retreatslive.com.

Contact me, Tom Woloshyn, for advanced cleansing and personal health coaching by email at tom@vitagem.com or by phone at (250) 388-4102.

Water Bottles

Good, stainless-steel water bottles are available at your local health food store and online at sites like www.healthyhome.com and www.greenfeet.com.

Offsetting Your Carbon Footprint

There are plenty of good websites to assist you in offsetting your carbon footprint. Trustworthy sites include: www.terrapass.com, www.renewablechoice.com and www.3phases.com.

Essential Oils

For information on how to obtain or use essential oils, my website, www.vitagem.com, is a great place to start.

Water Systems

Having good, clean, alkaline-balanced water is essential. I use the water alkalizer-ionizer manufactured by Life Ionizer (www.lifeionizer.com/lifemastercleanse).

Home and Body Products

There are many good sources for home and body products that are designed to be both healthy for you and for the planet. Two good sources for such items are www.momentum98.com and www.lovingtheplanet.com. To ensure that the body products you are using are healthy for you to use, go to the website www.cosmeticsdatabase.com.

For Further Reading

Burroughs, Stanley. *Healing for the Age of Enlightenment*. Reno, Nevada: Burroughs Books, 1976.

Emoto, Masaru. *The Hidden Messages in Water*. Hillsboro, Oregon: Beyond Words Publishing, 2004.

Foundation for Inner Peace. *A Course in Miracles*. Mill Valley, California: Foundation for Inner Peace, 1975.

Freston, Kathy. *Quantum Wellness: A Practical and Spiritual Guide to Health and Happiness*. New York: Weinstein Books, 2008.

Hay, Louise L. *You Can Heal Your Life*. Carson, California: Hay House, 1984.

Horn, Greg. *Living Green: A Practical Guide to Simple Sustainability*. Topanga, California: Freedom Press, 2006.

McCauley, Bob. *The Miraculous Properties of Ionized Water: The Definitive Guide to the World's Healthiest Substance*. Spartan Enterprises, Inc., 2006.

Pollan, Michael. *The Omnivore's Dilemma: A Natural History of Four Meals*. New York: Penguin Press, 2006.

Roy, Sondra. *I Deserve Love: How Affirmations Can Guide You to Personal Fulfillment*. Celestial Arts, 1976.

Tolle, Eckhart. *A New Earth: Awakening to Your Life's Purpose*. New York: Penguin Group, 2005.

Williamson, Marianne. *The Gift of Change: Spiritual Guidance for Living Your Best Life*. San Francisco: Harper, 2004.

Williamson, Marianne. *A Return to Love: Reflections on the Principles of "A Course in Miracles."* San Francisco: Harper, 1996.

Young, Robert O. and Shelley Redford Young. *The pH Miracle: Balance your Diet, Reclaim Your Health*. New York: Warner Books, 2003.

Index

Aknowledgments

To begin, I would like thank and dedicate this book to my friend, Robert Veal Jr., who was sadly killed in a motorcycle accident shortly after I completed my first book. His testimonial, which was included in that book, shattered many conventional beliefs about the Master Cleanse. Robert was a student of my work as well as a friend. He had a broad smile and a joy for life that is dearly missed by all who knew him.

I would also like to thank my friends and family for all their support over the many years as they have indulged me in discussing the Master Cleanse and other related topics. Thank you Adia, Kai, Shannon and Tamara.

Thank you to the many clients and students who have allowed me to learn and grow in this field and become a more proficient practitioner. You are the reason I love my work.

Thank you to the staff of Ulysses Press for editing, typesetting and publishing this book.

Stanley Burroughs, the original creator of the Master Cleanse, cannot be overlooked for his commitment to bringing a simple, yet profound system of healing to the planet. I will be forever indebted to him.

Finally, thank you to the Creative Power that makes all things possible.

About the Author

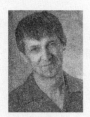

Tom Woloshyn began practicing and counseling in holistic health methods in 1980, after taking a course in the healing techniques of Stanley Burroughs. His main focus of expertise includes the following modalities: the Master Cleanse, Color Therapy, colon lifts, Vita-Flex massage, the mind–body connection, detoxification and the use of essential oils. He maintains a holistic health practice in Victoria, British Columbia, Canada.

Over the last 25 years Woloshyn has expanded his knowledge by working with a variety of teachers, including Burroughs himself, as well as by treating thousands of individuals. To share what he has learned, he has lectured and led workshops all around the world. He has also produced a DVD program, titled "Vita-Flex: The Instructional Video with Tom Woloshyn," that demonstrates the correct use of the technique. In order to share his expertise, Tom authored his first book, *The Complete Master Cleanse: A Step-by-Step Guide to Maximizing the Benefits of The Lemonade Diet.*

He is deeply committed to providing individuals the opportunity to better understand the body and the healing process, and to improve their own health and lives. He believes that, when people are given enough information, they will choose the proper path to wellness.

Tom Woloshyn welcomes inquiries and feedback. He can be contacted via his website, www.vitagem.com, or by telephone at (250) 388-4102 (please call after 9 a.m., Pacific time).